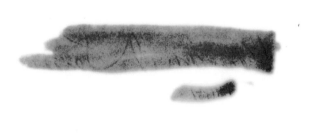

STEROID HORMONES
AND METABOLISM

PERSPECTIVES IN CELL BIOLOGY

a series of monographs
by KENNETH W. McKERNS

STEROID HORMONES
AND METABOLISM

Kenneth W. McKerns, Ph.D.

Professor, Department of Obstetrics and Gynecology, University of Florida College of Medicine, Gainesville

APPLETON-CENTURY-CROFTS

Educational Division

MEREDITH CORPORATION

NEW YORK

PRINTED IN THE UNITED STATES OF AMERICA

390-62298-2

To my wife, Dorothy,
who gave not only encouragement
but much practical assistance as well.

PREFACE

The average textbook of biochemistry is likely to be a dictionary or encyclopedia of reactions and molecular structures. The relevance of much of the material is not always clear to the beginning student or to the physician or others whose major field of interest has not been biochemistry and who might wish to learn modern concepts of cellular biochemistry.

It is tiresome to the student to study biochemistry simply by considering all of the possible enzymatic reactions that can occur in cells without knowing which are important in specialized cells. It is essential that some direction and significance be given to the study of processes that regulate the function of a cell. This monograph is therefore not a textbook in the usual sense. It attempts to explain fundamental aspects of molecular biochemistry and the regulation of cellular processes. The goal has been to present the necessary basic concepts and to develop them in terms of current ideas of regulation and function. The subject matter deals with the biosynthesis of steroid hormones and with certain control functions that these steroids have on cellular metabolism. Other hormones are considered where they have an influence on the organ or process under study. For example, when describing the effects of the glucocorticoids on the synthesis of glucose in the liver it was felt necessary to describe the action of other hormones such as insulin and epinephrine which can modify liver function.

The treatment of metabolic pathways has been in relation to specialized organs. Although some enzymes are shared in the two processes, gluconeogenesis needs to be understood as not just the reverse of glycolysis or the reverse of the effect of insulin in stimulating the metabolism of glucose by glycolysis. Glycolysis and gluconeogensis have been explained in reference to glucose homeostasis in the liver. It is expected that this could provide a working understanding of glycolysis in tissues such as muscle, brain, and adipose when conditions unique to each of these tissues are studied. Similarly, another major pathway for the metabolism of glucose by the pentose phosphate pathway is explained with special reference to the adrenal cortex. An understanding of glucose metabolism by this pathway as it occurs in liver, adipose, and other tissues can then be deduced. Lipid metabolism and its regulation are described in relation to metabolism in adipose tissue and to some aspects of liver function. The particular tissues treated as models for the definition of these processes were chosen because the regulatory effects of hormones have been studied extensively in them and are therefore better understood.

Genetic mechanisms in the control of cell function and growth have been developed in a general sense in regard to DNA replication and RNA and protein synthesis. Principles in the mechanism of action of hormones are related to genetic and metabolic processes. The steroid chemistry of the endocrines, biosynthesis of steroids, the mechanisms by which this is controlled, and some effects of steroids on target tissues have been described. Where possible the association of metabolism to function has been considered.

The control of function is influenced by enzymes that can convert substrates primarily in one direction. Thus, a metabolic pathway is established for the utilization of substrates for unique metabolic processes. The availability of substrates, the redox state of pyrimidine nucleotides, the variable rates of synthesis of certain enzymes, as well as the regulation of their activity, are all factors in determining cell function. Hormones are probably the ultimate regulators of metabolic processes in most mammalian cells. They regulate by inhibiting or stimulating activity or by inducing or suppressing the synthesis of enzymes, as well as influencing the availability of substrates in some cases.

By considering metabolic organization and control in the manner outlined, it is hoped that a great deal of molecular biology has been made understandable. Bibliographic references are to review articles as far as possible. These are supplemented by journal references where certain new ideas are not described in the review articles. They are provided as an introduction to further reading with no attempt made to assign priority or originality to authors.

A number of my colleagues were kind enough to read chapters of the monograph relative to their own areas of competence and to make helpful suggestions. For this I wish to thank Samuel H. Boyer, Isadore S. Edelman, Ronald W. Estabrook, David Fukushima, Hans A. Krebs, Paul D. Ray, Evan R. Simpson, Salih J. Wakil, and Abraham White.

Several others contributed. My wife Dorothy was of great assistance in the rewriting of the rough drafts to the final manuscripts. Mrs. Margaret Marsden conscientiously typed and retyped the manuscripts and assisted in the preparation of the index. Miss Glennda Whitehurst drew the diagrams from my rough sketches. Photographs of the drawings were made by the photography section of the Department of Medical Illustrations, Shands Teaching Hospital. Mrs. Patricia Wisler was of invaluable assistance in the writing of the chapter "Lipid Metabolism and Its Regulation."

Gainesville, Fla.
May 1969

Kenneth W. McKerns

CONTENTS

STEROID HORMONES
AND METABOLISM

1

Steroid Chemistry

Steroids such as androgen, estrogen, progesterone, and the corticoid hormones are derived from cholesterol. The synthesis of cholesterol has been discussed by Bloch and by Olson; the biosynthesis of various steroids from cholesterol is described in detail in the subsequent chapters of this book. Only some of the elementary aspects of the chemistry of the steroids will be considered here.

Carbon "rings" are the basic components of the steroid compounds to be described. A simple hexagon is used to represent a cyclohexane ring, and a benzene ring is indicated with three double bonds. As shown in Figure 1, each angle represents a carbon atom, and methyl groups are shown by straight lines. Hydrogen atoms are shown only where necessary—i.e., at the ends of straight lines not occupied by methyl groups.

In an attempt to achieve a three-dimensional representation of the molecules on paper, imagine that the plane of the ring systems corresponds to the surface of the paper. At asymmetric carbon atoms, position is specified by the number of the carbon atom, and orientation of the substituents by α or β. Hydrogen atoms or other substituents above the plane of the ring systems are β, indicated by a full-line bond; and substituents lying below the general plane of the ring system are α,indicated by dashed lines. For example, the angular methyl group (C-19) at C-10 position is β-oriented (Fig. 1).

In the cholesterol molecule, three six-carbon rings are fused with a five-carbon ring. This ring system is numbered A, B, C, and D, and is common to all the steroids (Fig.1). The structure of cholesterol is shown in Figure 2. The carbon atoms are numbered as shown. The hydroxyl group at C-3, the methyl groups at C-10 and C-13, as well as the side chain at C-17, are β-oriented, or above the plane of the ring system. The hydrogen atoms at C-3, C-9, C-14, and C-17 are α-oriented, relative to the plane of the ring system. The complete side chain at the C-17 position is above the plane of the ring system. This means that C-20 substituents have orientations within the new plane. The C-21 methyl group is used as the reference group and is given the rearmost position behind the C-20. (For convenience in the figure it is drawn to the left.) The C-20 hydrogen is actually to the left of the C-21 methyl and is called β. The isohexyl group on the right is α within the side chain. The convention of S and R designations can be used at this position to avoid confusion with the previous use of α and β, but steroid biochemists seldom employ it.

In addition to the spatial arrangements at the asymmetric centers, with configuration designated as α or β, there are conformational relationships in the rings of the steroid molecule. The rings are not planar, and cyclohexane can exist in two steric forms—the more thermodynamically stable chair form, and the boat form, as shown in Figure 3.

In the steroid hormone molecules, the rings are "fused" or are sharing common carbons at the 5-10, 8-9, and 13-14 positions. Since the carbons at these positions carry substituents which are either α or β, the rings can have a

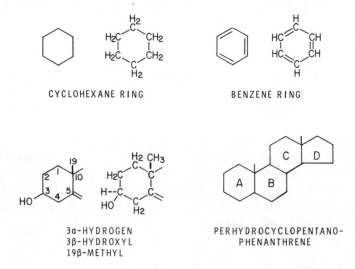

CYCLOHEXANE RING   BENZENE RING

3α-HYDROGEN   PERHYDROCYCLOPENTANO-
3β-HYDROXYL   PHENANTHRENE
19β-METHYL

Fig. 1. Representation of structure in steroid chemistry showing the cyclohexane ring, benzene ring, and perhydrocyclopentanophenanthrene. The last compound is the parent nucleus of steroid hormones.

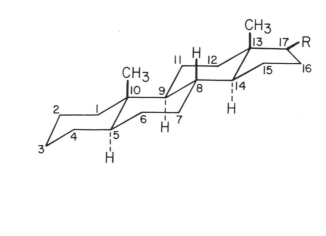

Fig. 2. The structure of cholesterol and the numbering of the carbon atoms.

"*cis*" or a "*trans*" relationship. In a *cis* relationship both the substituents are above the plane of the rings system, and in the *trans*, they are on opposite planes.

In the natural steroids, rings B and C are *trans* fused, in that the hydrogen atom at C-8 is β-oriented and at C-9 α-oriented. Rings C and D are also usually *trans* fused with the methyl group at C-13 β-oriented, and H at C-14 α-oriented. Most of the hormonally active steroids have a double bond between carbons 4 and 5. There is therefore no hydrogen at the C-5 position, and thus there is no *cis* or *trans* relationship to the β methyl group at C-10. When the 4-5 double

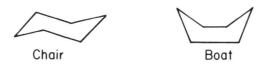

Chair   Boat

Fig. 3. Chair and boat forms of cyclohexane. The *trans* relationships between substituents at ring juctions 5-10, 8-9, and 13-14 in natural steroids are also shown, with cyclohexane rings in the chair form.

bond of the steroid hormone is reduced, as occurs in liver catabolism, the H at C-5 may lie on the same side of the molecule as the methyl at C-10 (A/B *cis*) or on the opposite side (A/B *trans*). The structure of relationships which are all *trans* between substituents at ring junctions 5-10, 8-9, and 13-14 is illustrated in Figure 3 with chair forms of the cyclohexane rings.

The naturally occurring steroids of human endocrine glands fall into three general classes represented by their reduced forms: pregnane, androstane, and estrane. These are shown in Figure 4. Systematic names for many of the naturally occurring steroids are given in Table 1.

Table 1. COMMON AND SYSTEMATIC NAMES OF CERTAIN NATURALLY OCCURRING STEROIDS

Common Name	Systematic Name
Cholestane	
Cholesterol	5-Cholesten-3β-ol
20α-Hydroxycholesterol	5-Cholestene-3β,20α-diol
20α,22ξ-Dihydroxycholesterol	5-Cholestene-3β,20α,22ξ-triol
Pregnane	
Pregnenolone	3β-Hydroxy-5-pregnen-20-one
17α-Hydroxypregnenolone	3β,17α-Dihydroxy-5-pregnen-20-one
Progesterone	4-Pregnene-3,20-dione
11α-Hydroxyprogesterone	11α-Hydroxy-4-pregnene-3,20-dione
17α-Hydroxyprogesterone	17α-Hydroxy-4-pregnene-3,20-dione
Corticosterone	11β,21-Dihydroxy-4-pregnene-3,20-dione
17α-Hydroxycorticosterone	11β,17α,21-Trihydroxy-4-pregnene-3,20-dione
11-Deoxycorticosterone	21-Hydroxy-4-pregnene-3,20-dione
18-Hydroxycorticosterone	11β,18,21-Trihydroxy-4-pregnene-3-20-dione
Aldosterone	3,20-Diketo-11β,21-dihydroxy-4-pregnen-18-al
Androstane	
Androstenedione	4-Androstene-3,17-dione
Dehydroepiandrosterone (dehydroisoandrosterone)	3β-Hydroxy-5-androsten-17-one
16α-Hydroxydehydroepiandrosterone	3β,16α-Dihydroxy-5-androsten-17-one
Testosterone	17β-Hydroxy-4-androsten-3-one
Estrane	
Estrone	3-Hydroxy-1,3,5(10)-estratrien-17-one
Estradiol	1,3,5(10)-Estratriene-3,17β-diol
Estriol	1,3,5(10)-Estratriene-3,16α,17β-triol

Fig. 4. The parent compounds of the three general classes of naturally occurring steroids: pregnane, androstane, and estrane.

PREGNANE (C_{21}) (CORTICOIDS)

ANDROSTANE (C_{19}) (ANDROGENS)

ESTRANE (C_{18}) (ESTROGENS)

A diagram representing various structures of a typical steroid-secreting cell is given in Figure 5. A more detailed description of the fine structure of steroid-secreting cells has been given by Christensen and associates (1969).

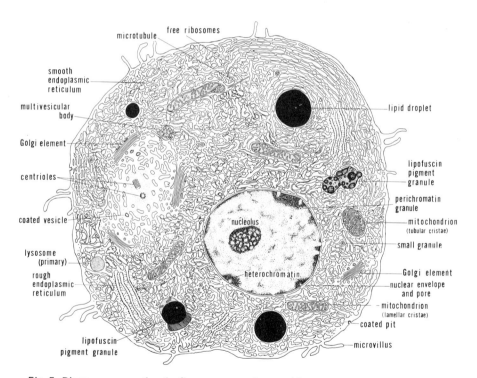

Fig. 5. Diagram representing the fine structures of a steroid-secreting cell. The mitochondria are characterized by tubular cristae. The large amount of smooth endoplasmic reticulum is actually a meshwork of interconnected tubules throughout the cytoplasm. The reticulum is drawn as it appears in electron micrographs of thin sections where tubules are cut and appear discontinuous. (From Christensen. *In* McKerns, ed. *The Gonads.* Appleton-Century-Crofts, 1969.)

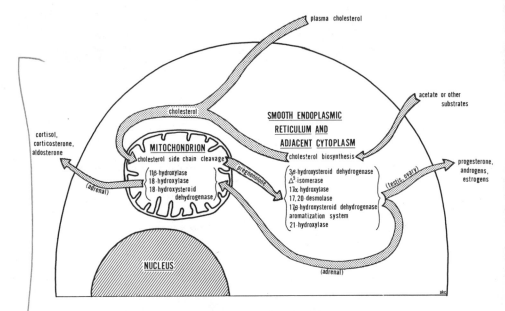

Fig. 6. This diagram shows the possible routes of steroid substances during hormone synthesis. Cholesterol may be derived from the plasma or synthesized in the smooth endoplasmic reticulum or cytoplasm. The side chain of cholesterol is cleaved in the mitochondrion, giving rise to pregnenolone. Pregnenolone is then transformed to other steroids in the reticulum or cytoplasm, depending on the particular endocrine organ. For example, in the adrenal cortex, pregnenolone is converted to progesterone by 3β-hydroxysteroid dehydrogenase and Δ^5-isomerase. Progesterone then can be converted to corticosterone by 21-hydroxylation in the reticulum and 11-hydroxylation in the mitochondria. Aldosterone can be formed from corticosterone in the mitochondria by 18-hydroxylase and 18-hydroxysteroid dehydrogenase. These and other reactions will be explained in various chapters. (From Christensen. *In* McKerns, ed. *The Gonads.* Appleton-Century-Crofts, 1969.)

Figure 6 illustrates the transformation of cholesterol to various steroids that can occur in structures in the cell. The type of steroid hormones that are synthesized—whether estrogen, androgen, progesterone, or corticoid—depends upon the presence and activity of special enzymes in the endocrine tissues. Reactions occurring in the steroid-secreting endocrines are given in detail in succeeding chapters of this book.

BLOCH, K. The biological synthesis of cholesterol. *Science*, 150:19, 1965.
CHRISTENSEN, A.K. and GILLIM, S.W. The correlation of fine structure and function in steroid-secreting cells, with emphasis on those of the gonads. *In* McKerns, K.W., ed. *The Gonads.* Part 2: Steroid-Secreting Cells. New York, Appleton-Century-Crofts, 1969, Chap. 16.
DORFMAN, R.I., and UNGAR, F. *Metabolism of Steroid Hormones.* New York, Academic Press, 1965.

FIESER, L.F., and FIESER, M. *Steroids*. New York, Reinhold Publishing Corp., 1959.

HEFTMAN, E., and MOSETTIG, E. *Biochemistry of Steroids*. New York, Reinhold Publishing Corp., 1960.

KLYNE, W. *The Chemistry of the Steroids*. London, Methuen & Co., Ltd., 1957.

OLSON, J.A. The biosynthesis of cholesterol. *Ergebn Physiol*, 56:173, 1965.

SHOPPEE, C.W. *Chemistry of the Steroids*. New York, Academic Press, 1958.

2

Steroidogenesis and Metabolism in the Adrenal Cortex

Many of the principles of steroid biochemistry can be learned from a study of the pathways of biosynthesis and the regulation of steroid hormones in the adrenal cortex because these are representative of what occurs in all endocrines that synthesize steroids. The mechanisms of electron transport in the mitochondria and microsomes that couple to reactions for the synthesis of steroids, as well as the source of electrons, are similar in steroid-secreting endocrines. In addition, mitochondria of the adrenal cortex have the "classical" electron-transport sequence, common to mitochondria of all tissues, whereby electrons derived from substrate oxidation are incorporated into high-energy bonds such as those of adenosine triphosphate.

PATHWAYS OF STEROIDOGENESIS

The adrenal cortex consists of three different zones of cells, each having different functions in terms of their hormone secretory products. These three

9

zones are the glomerular, under the capsule or outer membrane, followed by the fascicular and reticular zones. The particular steroid secretions of the various cellular layers of the adrenal cortex are determined by the spectrum of enzymes found in the various cell types. Thus, the potential hormone pattern secreted by these cell types is genetically determined. The expression of this genetic potential is controlled by various other regulating hormones, such as adrenocorticotropic hormone (ACTH), which we will consider later. The outer layer of the cortex, or glomerular zone, produces aldosterone, which is the principal steroid concerned in sodium reabsorption from the kidney tubule. ACTH stimulates pathways of steroidogenesis in the glomeruler zone from cholesterol to progesterones and corticosterones. Subsequent transformations of corticosterone to aldosterone are controlled largely by other mechanisms that will be considered later.

The fascicular-reticular border zone is markedly under the influence of ACTH. ACTH stimulates both cellular replication in these zones and the synthesis of glucocorticoids, such as 17α-hydroxycorticosterone and corticosterone. The reticular zone is the principal site of secretion of androgens such as androstenedione and dehydroepiandrosterone and, to a small extent, estrogens. When stimulated by ACTH, the fascicular-reticular zone of the adrenal cortex is able to transform cholesterol via a series of reactions to the final secretory products—glucocorticoids, androgens, and estrogens.

Many of these reactions are hydroxylation reactions carried out by specific hydroxylase enzymes that are coupled to electron-transport mechanisms in the mitochondria and microsomes for the activation and introduction of oxygen to form hydroxyl groups. The hydroxylase enzymes have a specific requirement for reducing equivalents (hydrogen) from the hydrogen carrier, NADPH (reduced nicotinamide adenine dinucleotide phosphate). Thus, the introduction of an atom of oxygen into the steroid molecule is concomitant with the oxidation of NADPH. The position on the steroid where molecular oxygen is introduced (C-11, C-21, etc.) is probably determined by the hydroxylase enzyme. The stoichiometry of these hydroxylation reactions may be written as

$$NADPH + H^+ + AH_2 + O{:}O \longrightarrow NADP^+ + AHOH + H_2O$$

The AH_2 represents the position on the steroid molecule where oxygen is introduced by the hydroxylase enzyme. There is evidence that the reducing equivalents come either directly from NADPH generated by enzymes of the pentose phosphate pathway, or from reverse electron flow in the metabolism of certain citric acid cycle substrates in the mitochondria such as isocitrate, α-ketoglutarate, or succinate. The relative importance of these two possible pathways of electron transport, their coupling to steroid hydroxylation reactions, and their possible competition with the synthesis of ATP in the mitochondria will be discussed in detail later in this chapter.

Reducing equivalents from NADPH are also required for hydroxylation and reductive reactions in the microsomes. Reduction of NADP$^+$ for this purpose is carried out by the metabolism of glucose-6-phosphate by glucose-6-phosphate dehydrogenase in the pentose phosphate cycle or by other NADP$^+$-specific dehydrogenases, such as isocitrate dehydrogenase. First the transformations of cholesterol through to final secretory products should be considered.

Steroid Synthesis in the Fascicular Zone

Some cholesterol is found in adrenal mitochondria, but more of it is found as lipid inclusions in the cytoplasm. In the cytoplasm, cholesterol is in the form of esters with fatty acids, such as palmitic acid, at the 3 position of cholesterol.

Let us examine in detail the transformation of cholesterol to 5-pregnenolone. This is carried out by a series of enzymes found in the mitochondria. The reaction sequence is indicated in Figure 1. The first reaction is the formation of a 20α-hydroxyl in the side chain of the cholesterol molecule by a specific

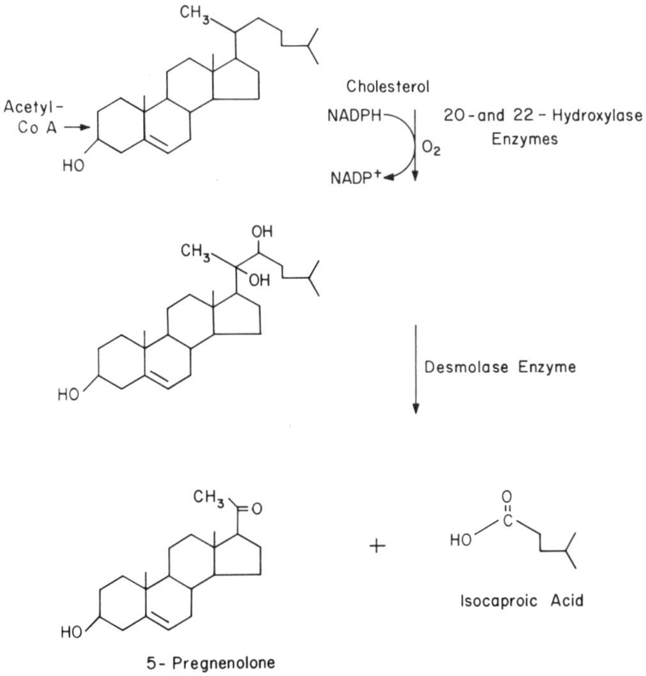

Fig. 1. Formation of 5-pregnenolone from cholesterol, via hydroxylations at the 20 and 22 positions on the sidechain to give 20α-22ξ-dihydroxycholesterol, with cleavage of the sidechain between C-20 and C-22. The orientation of the 22-hydroxyl is unknown (ξ). These reactions occur in the mitochondria. The hydroxylase enzymes require reducing equivalents from NADPH for introduction of molecular oxygen to form the hydroxyl group.

20α-hydroxylase enzyme. This would seem to be one of the slowest reactions in all of steroid transformations. It is followed rapidly by hydroxylation at the 22 position and a cleavage between these hydroxyl groups at the 20 and 22 positions by a desmolase enzyme. This yields 5-pregnenolone and isocaproic aldehyde, which is converted to isocaproic acid. The reaction sequence

$$\text{cholesterol} \longrightarrow 20\alpha\text{-hydroxycholesterol} \longrightarrow$$
$$20\alpha, 22\xi\text{-dihydroxycholesterol} \longrightarrow 5\text{-pregnenolone}$$

in the mitochondria has been considered to be a principal site of regulation of steroidogenesis by ACTH. This and other possible mechanisms of action of ACTH will be discussed in detail later.

The sequence of enzymes concerned in the formation of 5-pregnenolone from cholesterol in the mitochondria can be stimulated by the metabolism of citric acid cycle substrates such as isocitrate, malate, and succinate, which generate reducing equivalents for the respiratory chain leading to steroid hydroxylation. The formation of pregnenolone from cholesterol or ester cholesterol can be stimulated also by an increased rate of reduction of $NADP^+$ generated from the glucose-6-phosphate dehydrogenase reaction, which can be stimulated by ACTH. The generation and coupling of reducing equivalents to mitochondrial and microsomal electron transport will be discussed later.

Pregnenolone and progesterone can undergo a series of additional reactions that are shown in Figure 2. Pregnenolone can be converted to progesterone in the mitochondria. The first reaction is the removal of two hydrogens from the -CHOH group at position 3 by a 3 β-hydroxysteroid dehydrogenase specific for pregnenolone, which uses NAD^+ as the hydrogen acceptor. Thus, the enzyme converts the 3-hydroxyl group to a 3-ketone. The NADH formed may be reoxidized in the mitochondrial electron-transport sequence. The next enzyme or enzyme sequence is called Δ^5-3-ketosteroid isomerase and results in the shift of the double bond from the 5 to the 4 position.

In addition to the formation of progesterone from pregnenolone in the mitochondria, enzymes outside of the mitochondria, in the microsomes or in the cytoplasm, are able to carry out these reactions. In the cytoplasm they are stimulated by the availability of pyruvate for the lactic dehydrogenase reaction. This cytoplasmic NAD^+-lactic dehydrogenase is very active in the direction $NADH + \text{pyruvate} \longrightarrow NAD^+ + \text{lactate}$. Thus in the reduction of NAD^+ by 3β-hydroxysteroid dehydrogenase, the NADH is rapidly reoxidized by lactic dehydrogenase. The formation of progesterone from 5-pregnenolone in soluble preparations from adrenal cortex can also be stimulated by low levels of estradiol.

Another reaction that can occur in the mitochondria is 11-hydroxylation of progesterone or deoxycorticosterone. The activity of this 11-hydroxylase enzyme is important because all of the glucocorticoid compounds are 11-hydroxy derivatives. An 11-deoxy compound, such as 11-deoxycorticos-

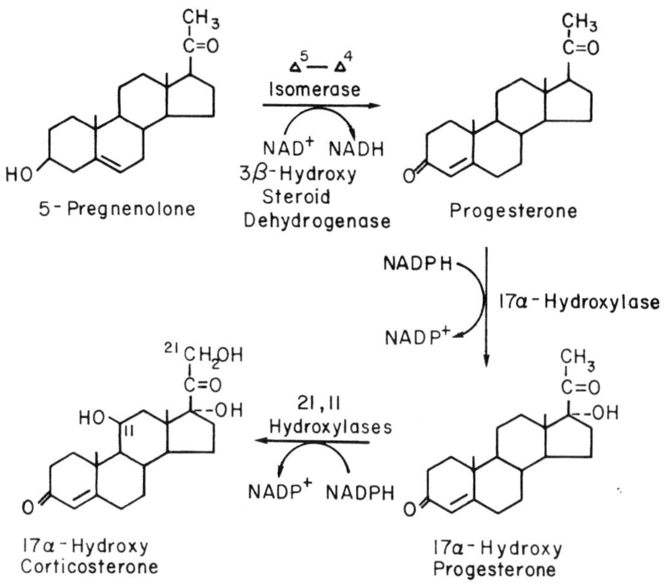

Fig. 2. Pathways in the formation of 17α-hydroxycorticosterone from 5-pregnenolone in the fascicular zone of the human adrenal cortex. The principal glucocorticoid is 17α-hydroxy-corticosterone (cortisol). Smaller amounts of corticosterone, which lacks a 17-hydroxyl, and deoxycorticosterone, which has neither a 17- nor 11-hydroxyl, are also secreted (see summary Fig. 8). Deoxycorticosterone is more active as a sodium-retaining compound than as a glucocorticoid.

terone, is more active as a sodium-retaining compound than as a glucocorticoid. The 17α-hydroxylase and 21-hydroxylase reactions occur outside the mitochondria. 21-Hydroxylation occurs largely in the microsomes of the endoplasmic reticulum, and 17α-hydroxylase activity is found both in soluble fractions and in the microsomes. If 11-hydroxyprogesterone is hydroxylated at the 17α and the 21 positions, it forms 17α-hydroxycorticosterone, the principal glucocorticoid of the human adrenal cortex. The series of reactions, 5-pregnenolone to 17α-hydroxycorticosterone, occurring in the fascicular zone is indicated in Figure 2. The principal secretory products of the fascicular zone in the human adrenal cortex are 17α-hydroxycorticosterone and, to a lesser extent, corticosterone (no 17-hydroxyl) and 11-deoxycorticosterone.

Steroid Synthesis in the Glomerular Zone

Aldosterone is synthesized in the glomerular zone. There are several possible pathways in the formation of this active sodium-retaining steroid. The principal pathways for the formation of aldosterone would seem to be the 21-hydroxylation of progesterone forming deoxycorticosterone, the 11-hydroxylation of this to give corticosterone, with subsequent 18-hydroxylation by

18-hydroxylase. The 18-hydroxy group would then be converted to an aldehyde by 18-ol-dehydrogenase, forming aldosterone. These pathways are indicated in Figure 3.

The conversion of the most likely precursor, corticosterone, to aldosterone occurs in the mitochondria. Hydroxylation at the C-18 position requires NADPH or the generation of reducing equivalents from citric acid cycle metabolites. The generation and utilization of reducing equivalents are described later in this chapter. In the conversion of 18-hydroxycorticosterone to aldosterone there

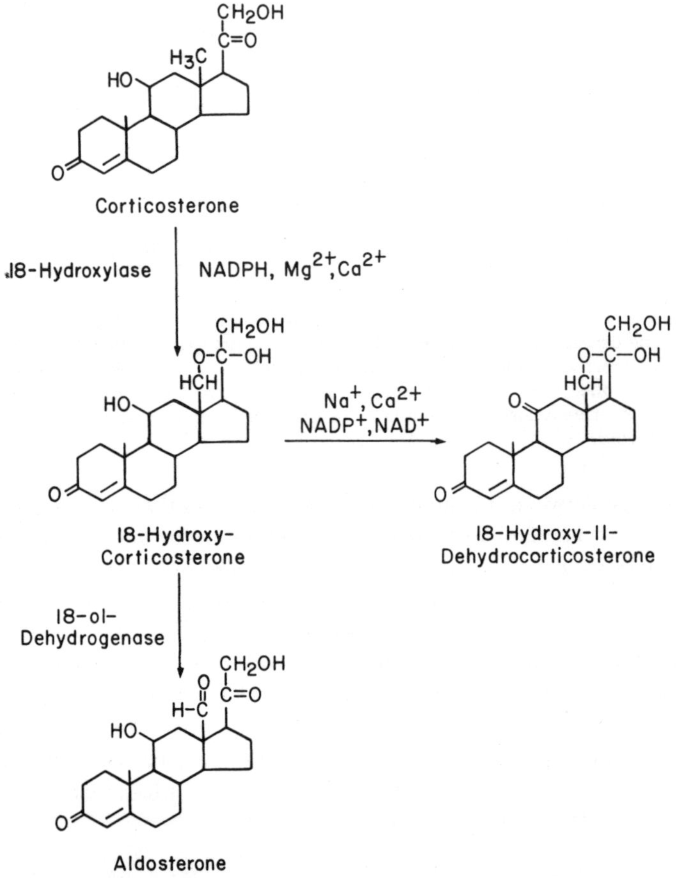

Fig. 3. Probable pathways in the formation of aldosterone from corticosterone in the glomerular zone of the adrenal cortex. The 18-hydroxylase enzyme requires reducing equivalents from NADPH. The 18-ol-dehydrogenase is able to form the aldehyde at the C-18 position, giving rise to aldosterone. These reactions, which are more complicated than indicated, occur in the mitochondria in the glomerular zone. A high concentration of sodium, in the presence of NAD^+ or $NADP^+$, may be able to stimulate directly the formation of 18-hydroxy-11-dehydrocorticosterone, which is less active than aldosterone as a sodium-retaining compound.

seems to be little effect of NADPH, but NAD^+ or $NADP^+$ stimulate the formation of 18-hydroxy-11-deoxycorticosterone and not aldosterone. There is also a Mg^{++} requirement for the synthesis of aldosterone and 18-hydroxycorticosterone. Mg^{++} can be replaced by Mn^{++} and to some extent by Ca^{++}. Na^+ has a stimulatory effect on the conversion of 18-hydroxycorticosterone into 18-hydroxy-11-deoxycorticosterone. This may represent a direct effect of Na^+ in decreasing the synthesis of aldosterone from 18-hydroxycorticosterone.

Steroid Synthesis in the Reticular Zone

Pregnenolone and progesterone are metabolized to androgens, as shown in Figure 4. Pregnenolone formed outside the mitochondria, or leaving the mitochondria, can be hydroxylated in a 17α configuration, forming 17α-hydroxypregnenolone. 17α-hydroxylase can be found in the soluble fraction from adrenal homogenates as well as in the microsomal fraction. The 17α side chain of the 17α-hydroxypregnenolone can be cleaved, leading to the formation of dehydroepiandrosterone. Dehydroepiandrosterone can be converted to androstenedione by a 3β-hydroxysteroid dehydrogenase enzyme specific for dehydroepiandrosterone, followed by an isomerase reaction.

Pregnenolone can also be converted by mitochondrial enzymes to progesterone, as shown in Figure 4. This is followed by 17α-hydroxylation.

The reticular zone is very active in the 17 side chain cleavage enzyme, which cleaves the side chain of 17α-hydroxypregnenolone or 17αhydroxyprogesterone to form androgens. The cleavage reactions which remove the 17 side chain and the isomerase enzyme are indicated in Figure 4, showing the formation of various androgens, mainly dehydroepiandrosterone and androstenedione in the reticular zone. To a limited extent these androgens may be converted to estrogens by aromatization reactions similar to those occurring in the ovary. These conversions are shown in Figure 5.

Sequence of Steroid Synthesis

The overall sequence of reactions in steroidogenesis that can occur in the three zones of the adrenal cortex and in other endocrine tissues is outlined in Figure 6. It should be kept in mind that quantitatively the principal secretions of the adrenal cortex are glucocorticoids, such as 17α-hydroxycorticosterones in the human and other species such as the cow. The rat adrenal lacks a 17α-hydroxylase enzyme, and the rat's prinicipal glucocorticoid is corticosterone. Lesser, but substantial amounts of compounds such as 11-deoxycorticosterone, androstenedione, and dehydroepiandrosterone are also secreted by the adrenal cortex. Aldosterone is a very potent mineralocorticoid, and thus is

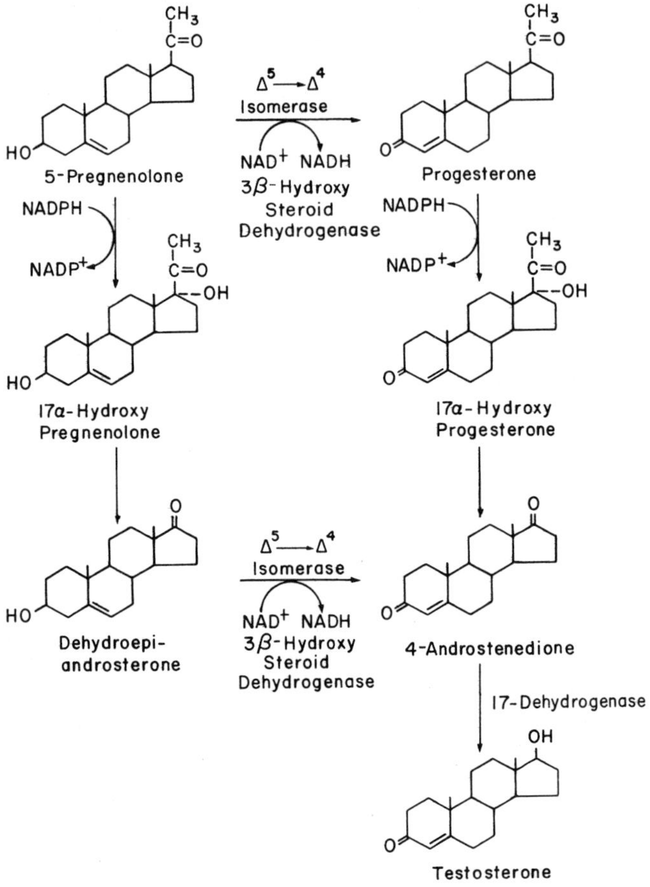

Fig. 4. Formation of androgens by the reticular zone of the adrenal cortex. These reactions are the same as those occurring in the Leydig cells of the testis. Androgens as precursors of estrogen formation in the follicular cells of the ovary are also synthesized by these pathways. 5-Pregnenolone, formed from cholesterol, is hydroxylated at the C-17 position in the microsomes. A side-chain cleavage or desmolase enzyme, also in the microsomes, removes the C-17 sidechain forming the 17-keto androgen, dehydroepiandrosterone. Much of the dehydroepiandrosterone is secreted. A specific 3β-hydroxysteroid dehydrogenase can form some of the corresponding 3-keto compound. Along with the isomerase reaction ($\Delta^5 \longrightarrow \Delta^4$) this leads to the formation of 4-androstenedione. Another route to 4-androstenedione is via the specific 3β-hydroxysteroid dehydrogenase for 5-pregnenolone, followed by the isomerase reaction giving progesterone. Progesterone is hydroxylated at the 17α-position, and desmolase cleavage of the 17 side chain gives 4-androstenedione. The two principal androgen secretory products of the adrenal cortex are, thus, dehydroepiandrosterone and 4-androstenedione. A small amount of testosterone may be formed from 4-androstenedione. Small amounts of the estrogen steroids, estrone and estradiol, can also be formed from androgens by aromatization reactions described in the chapter on the ovaries and shown in Figure 5.

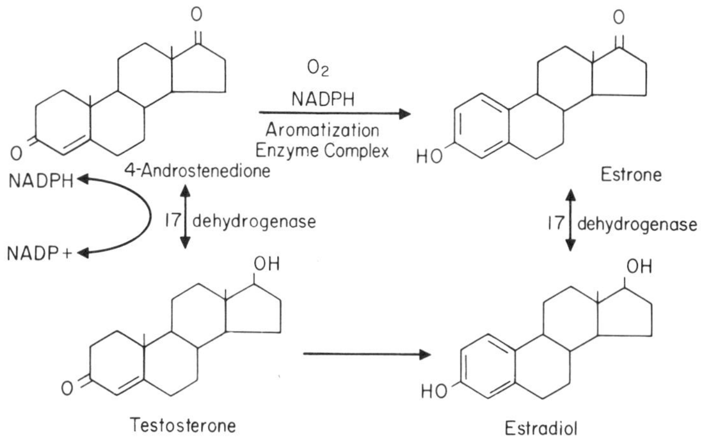

Fig. 5. Aromatization and the 17-dehydrogenase reactions of endocrine tissues that convert androgens to estrogens. These reactions require reducing equivalents from NADPH and occur to a limited extent in the adrenal cortex and possibly in the testis. They are more active in the granulosa cells of the ovarian follicle and in the placenta after the first trimester. The 17-dehydrogenase enzyme can reduce the 17-keto group with NADPH as the H-donor, or oxidize the 17α-hydroxyl with NADP$^+$ as H-acceptor. The aromatization-enzyme complex can form an estrogen corresponding to the androgen precursor.

produced usually only in small quantities, depending on the need for sodium reabsorption from the kidney tubules.

We now should consider the pathways of metabolites that yield electrons for the hydroxylation reactions, and in addition consider the pathways of electron flow in the mitochondria and microsomes. Possible mechanisms for the regulation of substrate metabolism and electron flow both for hydroxylations and reductions and for the synthesis of ATP will be discussed.

ENERGY METABOLISM IN THE ADRENAL CORTEX

It was mentioned earlier that the rate of reduction of NADP$^+$ is a major factor in the various hydroxylation and reductive reactions concerned in steroid synthesis. NADPH could be available to the steroid hydroxylation and reductive reactions through reduction of NADP$^+$ by the pentose phosphate pathway. Coupling of extramitochondrial NADPH to the mitochondrial steroid reactions may occur by way of a malate "shuttle," explained in the next section. The reduction of NADP$^+$ in the mitochondria could also occur by reverse electron flow from the metabolism of certain substrates of the citric acid cycle, such as isocitrate, α-ketoglutarate, or succinate, that reduce NAD$^+$ or FAD$^+$. These

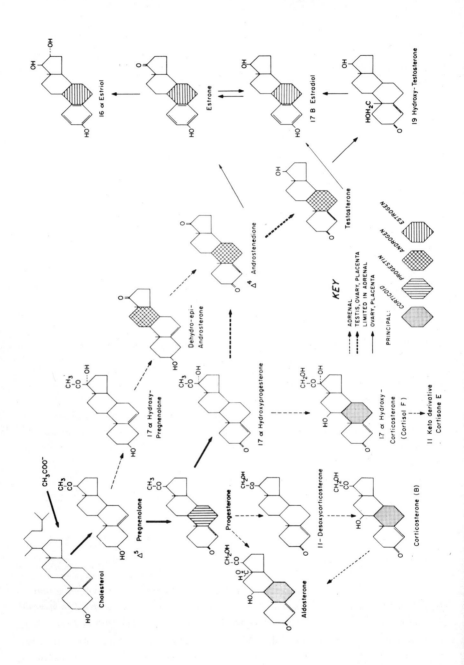

16 α Estriol

Estrone

17 B Estradiol

19 Hydroxy-Testosterone

Testosterone

Δ⁴ Androstenedione

Dehydro-epi-Androsterone

17 α Hydroxy-Pregnenolone

17 α Hydroxyprogesterone

17 α Hydroxy-Corticosterone (Cortisol F)

11 Keto derivative Cortisone E

CH₃COO⁻

Cholesterol

Δ⁵ Pregnenolone

Progesterone

11 - Desoxycorticosterone

Corticosterone (B)

Aldosterone

KEY

PRINCIPAL:
------ ADRENAL
–––– TESTIS, OVARY, PLACENTA
▪▪▪▪ LIMITED IN ADRENAL
⟶ OVARY, PLACENTA

ESTROGEN
ANDROGEN
PROGESTIN
CORTICOID

18

Fig. 6. Overall sequence of steroid synthesis occurring in the adrenal cortex and in other endocrine tissues that produce steroids. The principal types of steroids are indicated. Cholesterol is converted to 5-pregnenolone, then to progesterone and to mineralocorticoids such as aldosterone or 11-deoxycorticosterone, or to glucocorticoids such as corticosterone and 17α-hydroxycorticosterone in the adrenal cortex. The androgens dehydroepiandrosterone and 4-androstenedione are derived from 5-pregnenolore or progesterone, after 17α-hydroxylation and C-17 side-chain cleavage. These androgens are also secreted by the adrenal cortex, and along with testosterone they are the major secretory products of the adult testis. The follicles of the ovary further convert androgens to estrogens to form their major steroid-secretion products. The granulosa cells and the corpus luteum convert cholesterol to progesterones as their major steroid-secretion products. The fully developed placenta synthes zes progesterone from cholesterol as a secretory product, and converts androgens, brought to the placenta in the blood, to estrogens. Thus, the final secretory steroids are determined in each endocrine tissue by the spectrum and amount of various enzymes in their cells.

mechanisms will be explained later in the section on electron flow in the mitochondria and microsomes.

There are a number of possibilities for the mechanism of the action of ACTH in stimulating the production of reducing equivalents. Ideas concerning the mechanism of action of ACTH will be considered later, after a detailed examination of metabolic pathways of glucose-6-phosphate, metabolism of various substrates by the citric acid cycle of the mitochondria, and consideration of the electron-transport sequences in the mitochondria and microsomes.

There is no doubt that the metabolism of glucose is of prime importance to most tissues. However, the relative activities of the pentose phosphate pathway and glycolysis, the two main pathways for the metabolism of glucose, vary in different tissues. Glycolysis is discussed in the next chapter, on regulatory mechanisms of glucocorticoids. It is also outlined later in Figure 9 in this chapter. It is apparent that in all endocrine tissues the potential activity of the pentose phosphate pathway for the metabolism of glucose-6-phosphate is high. The regulation of the function of endocrines and some other tissues responsive to hormones may depend to a large extent on the control of the pentose phosphate pathway. This pathway seems to be the principal source of ribose sugars and their phosphorylated derivatives for the synthesis of nucleotides such as RNA. Thus, the pathway may be an active participant in the expression of the genetic potential of the cell. In other words, the availability of ribose sugars for synthesis of DNA and RNA may depend on this pathway. The pentose phosphate pathway is also of prime importance for the reduction of $NADP^+$ required for the synthesis of steroid hormones, as already mentioned. The pathway is undoubtedly important in adipose tissue metabolism and in lipid synthesis in many tissues. The rate of reduction of $NADP^+$ by this pathway, or its rate of utilization, may be rate-limiting in fatty acid synthesis. Glucose-6-phosphate is available for metabolism by the cell, either by the phosphorylation of glucose entering the cell or by the breakdown of stored glycogen. In the metabolism of glucose-6-phosphate by the pentose phosphate pathway the following factors are involved: the reduction of $NADP^+$, a cyclic possibility in the pathway, the formation of ribose sugars for nucleotide synthesis, and the capability to rejoin glycolysis at fructose-6-phosphate or glyceraldehyde-3-phosphate.

Metabolism of glucose-6-phosphate by the pentose phosphate pathway will now be considered in detail. The first enzymatic step involves the removal of two hydrogens (two protons plus two electrons) from C-1 of glucose-6-phosphate and the transfer of one hydrogen with an extra electron to position 4 of the nicotinamide moiety of $NADP^+$. A proton is released. This removal of two hydrogens from glucose-6-phosphate by the enzyme glucose-6-phosphate dehydrogenase gives rise to gluconolactone-6-phosphate, which is readily hydrolyzed to gluconate-6-phosphate by lactonase. The reduction of $NADP^+$ is shown in Figure 7. Various reactions of the pentose phosphate pathway are given in detail in Figure 8.

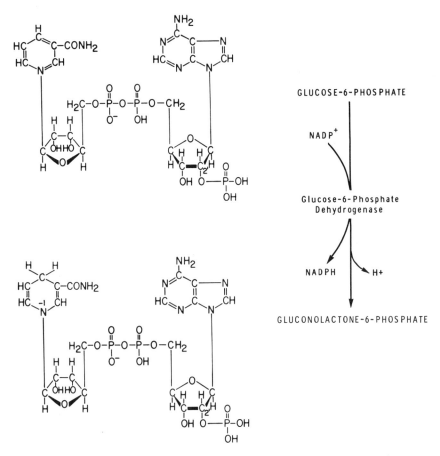

Fig. 7. The reduction of nicotinamide adenine dinucleotide phosphate (NADP$^+$) by the NADP$^+$-specific glucose-6-phosphate dehydrogenase reaction. Hydrogen (with an extra electron) is transferred from C-1 of glucose-6-phosphate to the pyridine ring of the coenzyme NADP$^+$. Associated with this is the release of a proton so that glucose-6-phosphate loses two hydrogens. Thus, the pyridine ring becomes reduced, retaining only two double bonds. NADP$^+$ can be considered as having a net charge of 0 and NADPH as -1. NADP$^+$ and NAD$^+$ (which lacks a phosphate group at the 2$'$-position) can accept hydrogen from a number of substrates by means of specific dehydrogenases. The other dehydrogenase in the pentose phosphate pathway is NADP$^+$-gluconate-6-phosphate dehydrogenase.

Next, 6-phosphogluconic acid is enzymatically decarboxylated, along with another transfer of hydrogen to NADP$^+$, yielding the pentose sugar D-ribulose-5-phosphate. This sugar in turn can give rise to ribose sugar phosphates, such as D-ribose-5-phosphate and 5-phospho-D-ribosyl pyrophosphate. These ribose sugars, as mentioned previously, are essential components in the synthesis of nucleotides. Their association to nucleotide synthesis is explained in the chapter on DNA, RNA, and protein synthesis and in the chapter on the mechanism of action of hormones. The pentose phosphate pathway can consist of a cyclic

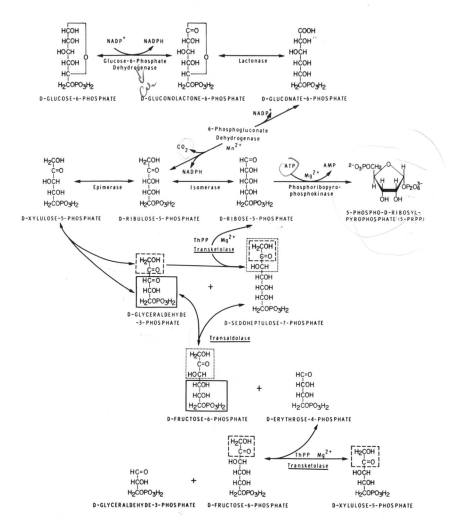

Fig. 8. This series of reactions outlines various possibilities in the metabolism of glucose-6-phosphate by the pentose phosphate pathway, also called the phosphogluconate oxidative pathway. These cytoplasmic enzymes have a high order of activity in endocrine tissues, mammary gland, adipose tissue, leukocytes, and liver. The pathway provides reducing equivalents as NADPH for steroid and fatty acid synthesis, and for reduction and detoxification processes of steroids and drugs in the liver. It also provides pentose sugars such as 5-phospho ribosyl pyrophosphate for nucleotide biosynthesis.

Glucose-6-phosphate dehydrogenase catalyzes the oxidation of glucose-6-phosphate to gluconolactone-6-phosphate, with the reduction of NADP$^+$. Gluconolactone-6-phosphate is hydrolyzed to the corresponding acid by a specific lactonase. Equilibrium for these reactions is far to the right. Glucose-6-phosphate is further oxidized, and another NADP$^+$ is reduced by 6-phosphogluconate dehydrogenase an oxidative decarboxylase. The decarboxylation and reduction yield ribulose-5-phosphate. This pentose sugar can be interconverted into two isomeric pentoses, xylulose-6-phosphate by an epimerase, or ribose-5-phosphate by an isomerase. Xylulose-5-phosphate is a source of "active glycoaldehyde" in the transketolase reaction. One example of this reversible reaction is the transfer of the 2-carbon unit system for the total metabolism of glucose-6-phosphate without requiring ATP. This is so because excess ribose sugars can rejoin the glycolytic pathway, either by way of fructose-6-phosphate or by way of D-glyceraldehyde-3-phosphate, as a result of the transaldolase or the transketolase reactions. Both fructose-6-phosphate and glyceraldehyde-3-phosphate, as well as recycling through the pentose phosphate pathway, could in addition be available for energy metabolism by way of glycolysis to pyruvate. This is indicated in Figure 9.

Glyceraldehyde-3-phosphate can be metabolized to pyruvate and, in the process, yields two molecules of ATP from two molecules of ADP as well as causes the reduction of one molecule of NAD^+. Pyruvate can form acetyl-CoA, condense with oxalacetate in the mitochondria to form citrate, and be oxidized by the citric acid cycle. Pyruvate can also form oxalacetate by the pyruvate carboxylase reaction (Chapter 3, Figure 10), or form malate via $NADP^+$-malate enzyme (Chapter 2, Figure 10). Electrons captured by various acceptors during metabolism of substrates can traverse the mitochondrial electron-transport sequences, either for ATP synthesis or for steroid hydroxylations.

The earlier steps of glycolysis for the metabolism of glucose-6-phosphate involve the formation of 1,6-diphosphate sugar and its splitting into two triose sugars that can yield two molecules of D-glyceraldehyde-3-phosphate. These and other reactions in glycolysis are given in detail in the next chapter. The association of glycolysis and the pentose phosphate pathway to mitochondrial function is also considered in Figure 9 in this chapter. A variety of other substrates, such as amino acids or fatty acids, may give rise to intermediates of the citric acid cycle or to substrates, such as α-glycerophosphate or β-hydroxy-butyrate, that may be oxidized directly in the mitochondria.

Fig. 8 (con't). from xylulose-5-phosphate to ribose-5-phosphate, forming the 7-carbon sugar sedoheptulose and glyceraldehyde-3-phosphate. Thiamine pyrophosphate (ThPP) is required as coenzyme, and the enzyme requires Mg^{++}.

Transaldolase can effect the transfer of carbon atoms 1 to 3 of a ketose phosphate, such as sedoheptulose, to C-1 of an aldose phosphate, such as glyceraldehyde-3-phosphate. In the transaldolase reaction shown, fructose-6-phosphate and erythrose-4-phosphate are formed. The erythrose-4-phosphate accepts a 2-carbon unit from xylulose-5-phosphate in another transketolase reaction to yield fructose-6-phosphate and glyceraldehyde-3-phosphate.

Glyceraldehyde-3-phosphate and fructose-6-phosphate formed by the transketolase-transaldolase reactions, described above, can reform glucose-6-phosphate with the following four enzymes. Triose isomerase interconverts glyceraldehyde-3-phosphate and dihydroxy-acetone phosphate. These two triose phosphates are catalyzed by fructoaldolase to form fructose-1,6-diphosphate. This latter compound is hydrolyzed by fructose-1,6-diphosphatase to fructose-6-phosphate. Phosphohexose isomerase converts fructose-6-phosphate to glu-cose-6-phosphate. The reactions of these four enzymes are described in Chapter 3, in the section on gluconeogenesis and glycolysis in the liver.

The oxidation of 6 moles of glucose-6-phosphate to ribulose-6-phosphate would result in the transfer of 12 electrons to $NADP^+$ (equal to the total oxidation of 1 mole of glucose to 6 moles of CO_2). This would leave 6 moles of ribulose-6-phosphate which could be isomerized to 6 moles of ribose-5-phosphate. If these are not converted to 5-phosphoribosyl pyrophosphate, they could be rearranged in the transketolase-transaldolase reactions for complete oxidation in the cycle as described.

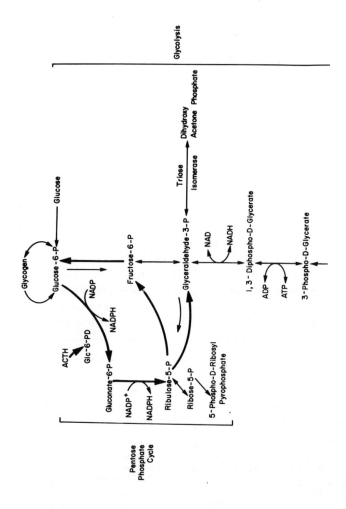

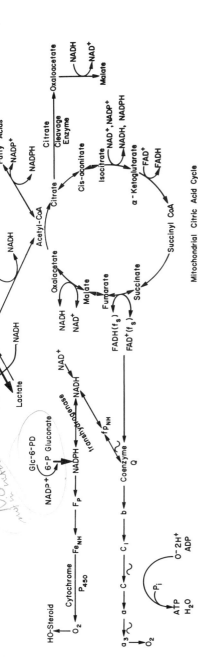

Mitochondrial Electron Transport

Mitochondrial Citric Acid Cycle

Fig. 9. The association of substrate oxidation to the synthesis of ATP and steroid hydroxylation in the adrenal cortex. The pentose phosphate pathway can form a cyclic system for the reduction of NADP⁺ and the metabolism of glucose-6-phosphate via ribulose-5-phosphate back to fructose-6-phosphate by reducing the apparent Km for both glucose-6-phosphate and NADP⁺. NADPH can couple to the steroid electron-transport chain shown in the upper line on the left side of the diagram. This introduction of reducing equivalents from NADPH into the mitochondria most likely occurs via malate, as explained in Figure 10.

The pentose phosphate cycle also provides ribose sugars such as 5-phospho-D-ribosyl pyrophosphate required in the synthesis of pyrimidines and purines required in RNA and other nucleotide synthesis.

Ribulose-5-phosphate not recycling to fructose-6-phosphate or forming ribose sugars can rejoin the glycolytic pathway at glyceraldehyde-3-phosphate. The glycolytic pathway provides some reducing equivalents in the form of NADH and some ATP, as indicated. The amount of glucose-6-phosphate metabolized entirely by glycolysis varies in different tissues. Pyruvate from the final steps of glycolysis is available for oxidation by the mitochondria via the formation of acetyl-CoA which condenses with oxalacetate to form citrate, or by formation of oxalacetate by the pyruvate carboxylase reaction. Citrate is oxidized through the enzyme reactions of the citric acid cycle with a reduction of NAD⁺ or FAD⁺. These two electron carriers couple to coenzyme Q, as indicated. Electrons are transported along the chain, enabling ADP with inorganic phosphate (Pi) to form the high-energy ATP indicated at three steps by ∼. H₂O is also formed. The proton remaining after the removal of electrons from hydrogen reacts with oxygen to form water, or the proton may leave the mitochondria with a corresponding translocation of other ions such as Ca⁺⁺ or Mg⁺⁺. Pyruvate also takes part in a shuttle system for trapping hydrogen from NADPH, as explained in Figure 10.

The two electron-transport chains may be bridged by an energy-dependent transhydrogenase enzyme between NADP⁺ and NAD⁺. However, ATP synthesis may couple largely to substrate oxidation in the mitochondrial citric acid cycle, whereas steroid hydroxylation probably couples largely to NADPH formed outside the mitochondria, as described previously, and in Figure 10.

ELECTRON FLOW IN THE MITOCHONDRIA AND MICROSOMES

Glycolysis can provide reducing equivalents. In the metabolism of glyceraldehyde-3-phosphate to 1,3-diphosphoglycerate and in the metabolism of pyruvate to acetyl-CoA, NAD^+ is reduced. These reducing equivalents (NADH) may be used for extramitochondrial reactions, or may possibly couple to intramitochondrial electron-transport chains. However, most, if not all, of the reducing equivalents donating electrons for the synthesis of ATP come from intramitochondrial reduction of NAD^+ or FAD by metabolism of substrates of the citric acid cycle. These substrates derived from pyruvate can be acetyl-CoA and oxalacetate, which condense to form citrate in the mitochondria. On the other hand, steroid hydroxylation is coupled to a unique electron-transport chain found in microsomes as well as mitochondria, which utilizes reducing equivalents from NADPH. As discussed earlier, NADPH is probably available mostly from the pentose phosphate pathway. However, it is also possible that a nonenergy-linked transhydrogenase exists in the cytoplasm to transfer reducing equivalents formed during glycolysis from NADH to $NADP^+$.

There are two pathways for electron transport in adrenal mitochondria, with a possible energy-dependent transhydrogenase linking the two electron-transport chains. These two pathways for electron transport are indicated in Figure 9, which also shows the coupling of reducing equivalents from the mitochondrial citric acid cycle and from the reduction of $NADP^+$ by extramitochondrial enzymes. These two chains for electron transport have unique functions. The classical electron-transport chain concerned in the removal of electrons from hydrogen for the synthesis of ATP from ADP is shown in the lower line on the left of Figure 9.

In metabolic reactions of the citric acid cycle, such as the conversion of succinate to fumarate, and α-ketoglutarate to succinyl-CoA, electrons are captured by the flavin adenine dinucleotide, $FAD^+(f_s)$, which passes electrons to coenzyme Q and through the cytochrome chain sequence b $\longrightarrow$ c_1 $\longrightarrow$ c $\longrightarrow$ a $\longrightarrow$ a_3 and to O_2. NAD^+ may be reduced in the mitochondria by reactions such as the conversion of isocitrate by NAD^+-isocitric dehydrogenase with the formation of NADH and α-ketoglutarate, or by the metabolism of malate to oxalacetate. NADH may enter the ATP-synthesizing chain via an NADH dehydrogenase which contains a nonheme iron flavoprotein (fp_{NH}). In the electron-transport chain, electrons may be transferred from FADH or NADH, with a formation of adenosine triphosphate (ATP) from ADP between fp_{NH} $\longrightarrow$ coenzyme Q, and between the cytochromes c_1 $\longrightarrow$ c, and a $\longrightarrow$ a_3. The formation of the high-energy compound ATP from ADP is indicated by the squiggle line ($\sim$). This occurs as a consequence of the capture by ADP and Pi of the energy lost by the electron in transferring from a higher energy compound to one of lower energy, as occurs at the three steps indicated.

The other electron-transport chain in the mitochondria is concerned with providing reducing equivalents required in steroid hydroxylation. This steroid-hydroxylating electron-transport chain is indicated in the upper line on the left of Figure 9. This electron-transport chain consists of NADPH $\longrightarrow$ flavoprotein (Fp) $\longrightarrow$ nonheme iron protein (Fe_{NH}) $\longrightarrow$ cytochrome P_{450} $\longrightarrow$ O_2. The unique cytochrome P_{450} couples with specific hydroxylases (mixed function oxidases) for the introduction of an atom of oxygen into the steroid molecule. $NADP^+$ reduced outside the mitochondria or on the mitochondrial membrane by enzymes of the pentose phosphate pathway can couple to the electron-transport chain for steroid hydroxylations occurring in the mitochondria, as will be explained later. In addition, reverse electron flow from NADH may be possible, as indicated in Figure 9. This consists of transfer of electrons from the mitochondrial citric acid cycle (such as may be generated by the oxidation of succinate) by way of coenzyme Q to fp_{NH} to mitochondrial NAD^+. An energy-dependent (ATP) transhydrogenase may exist for the exchange of electrons from NADH to $NADP^+$. By this mechanism $NADP^+$ could be reduced and electrons made available to the rest of the electron-transport sequence concerned in steroid hydroxylation. This would compete with the synthesis of ATP.

As mentioned, steroid reactions coupling to electron transport in the mitochondria consist of the 20 α-hydroxylase and the 22-hydroxylase enzymes, in the conversion of cholesterol to 5-pregnenolone, and the 11-hydroxylase enzyme. The 18-hydroxylation of corticosterone in the pathway to aldosterone in the glomerular zone also utilizes similar mechanisms for the reduction of $NADP^+$, along with a mixed function oxidase requiring NADPH, O_2, and involving cytochrome P_{450}.

The coupling of succinate oxidation in the citric acid cycle to the $NADP^+$-steroid electron-transport chain in the mitochondria may play a minor role. More important may be the reduction of $NADP^+$ outside the mitochondria by enzymes such as $NADP^+$-isocitrate dehydrogenase, and glucose-6-phosphate dehydrogenase and 6-phosphogluconate dehydrogenase of the pentose phosphate cycle. Oldham, Bell, and Harding have shown that the rate of hydroxylation supported by $NADP^+$-isocitrate dehydrogenase in adrenal mitochondria is considerably less than that supported by malate. Malate is a transport form of extramitochondrial reducing equivalents from NADPH, as we shall see later. Thus, reduction of $NADP^+$ by the pentose phosphate cycle may be the major source of reducing equivalents for mitochondrial hydroxylations, as well as for the extramitochondrial reactions in the microsomes and cytoplasm. ACTH can increase the rate of reduction of $NADP^+$ by the glucose-6-phosphate dehydrogenase reaction, especially at the cellular levels of $NADP^+$ and glucose-6-phosphate, and thus may be a major stimulator to reducing equivalents.

NADPH generated in the cytoplasm can efficiently couple to mitochondrial electron transport for steroid hydroxylation through the interaction of malate enzymes. Simpson, Cammer, and Estabrook have demonstrated the existence of two malic enzymes. A cytoplasmic malic enzyme was isolated from the bovine adrenal cortex with greater activity in the direction:

$$\text{pyruvate} + CO_2 + NADPH \longrightarrow \text{malate} + NADP^+$$

Thus, this enzyme has the capacity to fix carbon dioxide and take up reducing equivalents from extramitochondrial NADPH. Malate can then enter the mitochondria where it is oxidized by a different mitochondrial malate enzyme that has marked activity in the opposite direction. Pyruvate is reformed and intramitochondrial $NADP^+$ is reduced and available directly to the steroid hydroxylating chain. Péron and Caldwell have also described a possible malate shuttle as a mechanism for bringing reducing equivalents into the mitochondria. These reactions are illustrated in Figure 10.

ATP synthesis does not occur in the microsomes. The microsomes of the endoplasmic reticulum of the adrenal cortex and other endocrines that synthesize steroid hormones contain only a steroid electron-transport sequence. This electron-transport chain couples to 21-hydroxylase and probably 17α-hydroxylase reactions in corticoid synthesis. Aromatization reactions in the

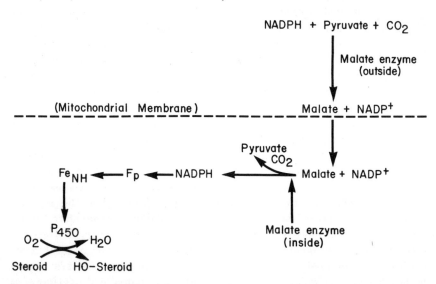

Fig. 10. The role of malate as a shuttle for carrying reducing equivalents from outside into the mitochondria for the $NADP^+$-steroid hydroxylating chain. Malate enzyme outside the mitochondria can fix carbon dioxide and take up reducing equivalents from NADPH to form malate. Malate enters the mitochondria, and the reverse reaction proceeds by an intramitochondrial malate enzyme. $NADP^+$ inside the mitochondria is thus reduced, and electrons are captured by the steroid hydroxylating chain.

conversion of androgens to estrogens also occur in the microsomes and require NADPH. The reduction of $NADP^+$ by enzymes of the pentose phosphate cycle would seem to be a principal source of electrons for these reactions.

The components of the electron-transport sequence in microsomes of steroid-synthesizing endocrines have not all been identified. Cooper and associates have studied the mechanism of C-21 hydroxylation of steroids such as progesterone and 17-hydroxyprogesterone in adrenocortical microsomes. These microsomes apparently contain two cytochrome-C reductase flavoproteins, one of which oxidizes NADPH. Atmospheric oxygen and NADPH are required by adrenocortical microsomes for 21-hydroxylation of steroids such as progesterone. Cytochrome P_{450} was identified as the oxidase of the steroid 21-hydroxylase system. This cytochrome requires electrons for the activation of oxygen which is introduced between the carbon at position 21 and one of the hydrogens. Specificity is probably achieved by the association of cytochrome P_{450} with a specific C-21 hydroxylase enzyme.

CAMMER, W., COOPER, D.Y., and ESTABROOK, D.W. Electron transport reactions for steroid hydroxylation by adrenal cortex mitochondria. *In* McKerns, K.W., ed. *Functions of the Adrenal Cortex*. New York, Appleton-Century-Crofts, 1968, Vol. 2, Chap. 24.

CHANCE, B. The reactivity of haemoproteins and cytochromes. *Biochem J*, 103:1, 1967.

COOPER, D.Y., NARASIMHULU, S., ROSENTHAL, O., and ESTABROOK, R.W. Studies on the mechanism of C-21 hydroxylation of steroids by the adrenal cortex. *In* McKerns, K.W., ed. *Functions of the Adrenal Cortex*. New York, Appleton-Century-Crofts, 1968, Vol. 2, Chap. 23.

CRISS, W.E. and McKERNS, K.W. Activation of cow adrenal glucose-6-phosphate dehydrogenase by adrenocorticotropin. *Biochemistry*, 7:2364, 1968.

GREEN, D.E. Structure and function of subcellular particles. *Comp Biochem Physiol*, 4:81, 1962.

GREENGARD, P., TALLAN, H.H., and PSYCHOYOS, S. Biosynthesis of aldosterone in cell free systems. *In* McKerns, K.W., ed. *Functions of the Adrenal Cortex*. New York, Appleton-Century-Crofts, 1968, Vol. 1, Chap. 7.

HALKERSTON, I.D. On the heterogeneity of the response of adrenal cortex tissue slices to adrenocorticotrophin. *In* McKerns, K.W., ed. *Functions of the Adrenal Cortex*. New York, Appleton-Century-Crofts, 1968, Vol. 1, Chap. 10.

HARDING, B.W., BELL, J.J., OLDHAM, S.B., and WILSON, L.D. Corticosteroid biosynthesis in adrenal cortical mitochondria. *In* McKerns, K.W., ed. *Functions of the Adrenal Cortex*. New York, Appleton-Century-Crofts, 1968, Vol. 2, Chap. 22.

ICHIKAWA, Y., YAMANO, T., and FUJISHIMA, H. Relationship between the interconversion of cytochrome P-450 and P-420 and its activities in hydroxylations and demethylations by P-450 oxidase systems. *Biochim Biophys Acta*, 171:32, 1969.

KIMURA, T. Electron transfer system of steroid hydroxylases in adrenal mitochondria. *In* McKerns, K.W., ed. *Functions of the Adrenal Cortex*. New York, Appleton-Century-Crofts, 1968, Vol. 2, Chap. 25.

KORITZ, S.B. On the regulation of pregnenolone synthesis. *In* McKerns, K.W., ed. *Functions of the Adrenal Cortex*. New York, Appleton-Century-Crofts, 1968, Vol. 1, Chap. 2.

McKERNS, K.W. Mechanisms of ACTH regulation of the adrenal cortex. *In* McKerns, K.W., ed. *Functions of the Adrenal Cortex*. New York, Appleton-Century-Crofts, 1968, Vol. 1, Chap. 12.

——Mechanism of action of adrenocorticotropic hormone through activation of glucose-6-phosphate dehydrogenase. *Biochim Biophys Acta*, 90:357, 1964.

OLDHAM, S.B., BELL, J.J., and HARDING, B.W. Role of the bovine adrenal cortical pyridine nucleotide transhydrogenase in steroid 11β-hydroxylation. *Arch Biochem*, 123:496, 1968.

PÉRON, F.G., and McCARTHY, J.L. Corticosteroidogenesis in the rat adrenal gland. *In* McKerns, K.W., ed. *Functions of the Adrenal Cortex*. New York, Appleton-Century-Crofts, 1968, Vol. 1, Chap. 8.

PÉRON, F.G., and CALDWELL, B.V. Further studies on corticosteroidogenesis. V. 11β-hydroxylation of DOC by mitochondria incubated with malate, supernatant fraction and supernatant fraction + pyruvate + CO_2. *Biochim Biophys Acta*, 164:396, 1968.

PURVIS, J.L., BATTU, R.G., and PÉRON, F.G. Generation and utilization of reducing power in the conversion of 11-deoxycorticosterone to corticosterone in rat adrenal mitochondria. *In* McKerns, K.W., ed. *Functions of the Adrenal Cortex*. New York, Appleton-Century-Crofts, 1968, Vol. 2, Chap. 26.

ROBERTS, S., and CREANGE, J.E. The role of 3',5'-adenosine phosphate in the subcellular localization of regulatory processes in corticosteroidogenesis. *In* McKerns, K.W., ed. *Functions of the Adrenal Cortex*. New York, Appleton-Century-Crofts, 1968, Vol. 1, Chap. 9.

SIMPSON, E.R., and BOYD, G.S. Studies on the conversion of cholesterol to pregnenolone in bovine adrenal mitochondria. *In* McKerns, K.W., ed. *Functions of the Adrenal Cortex*. New York, Appleton-Century-Crofts, 1968, Vol. 1, Chap. 3.

——, CAMMER, W., and ESTABROOK, R.W. The role of malic enzyme in bovine adrenal cortex mitochondria. *Biochem Biophys Res Commun*, 31:113, 1968.

——and ESTABROOK, R.W. Mitochondrial malic enzyme: The source of reduced nicotinamide adenine dinucleotide phosphate for steroid hydroxylation in bovine adrenal cortex mitochondria. *Arch Biochem Biophys*, 129:384, 1969.

TCHEN, T.T. Conversion of cholesterol to pregnenolone in the adrenal cortex; enzymology and regulation. *In* McKerns, K.W., ed. *Functions of the Adrenal Cortex*. New York, Appleton-Century Crofts, 1968, Vol. 1, Chap. 1.

3

Regulatory Mechanisms of Glucocorticoids and Associated Hormonal Changes

The glucocorticoid hormones of the adrenal cortex, such as cortisol, have several important functions in regulating cellular processes in the body. They are essential to the production of glucose from short-chain precursors by gluconeogenesis. In gluconeogenesis, glucocorticoids act to inhibit protein synthesis in peripheral tissue and thus release free amino acids from muscle and other tissues to the liver. In the liver these amino acids are converted by transamination and other reactions to pyruvate or oxalacetate and eventually to glucose. Nitrogen (NH_4^+) from amino acids is converted to urea by the liver. This synthesis of carbohydrate from pyruvate and oxalacetate is not a direct reversal of glycolysis, which is the process of metabolism of glucose to pyruvate or lactate. As will be seen later, several enzyme reactions are unique to gluconeogenesis and others are unique to the metabolism of glucose by glycolysis. Glucocorticoids also stimulate the breakdown of lipids in adipose tissue, resulting in the release of free fatty acids and glycerol. Epinephrine, which is released from the adrenal medulla, also has a role in the release of glycerol and free fatty acids from adipose tissue. Epinephrine does this by activating lipases. Glycerol is a precursor of glucose in the liver, whereas free fatty acids inhibit the utilization of glucose by the liver.

31

The important initial effects of glucocorticoids, then, are to increase amino acid precursors for the synthesis of glucose and, via an increase in free fatty acid from adipose tissue, to decrease the activity of enzymes concerned in the utilization of glucose. Other early, but apparently secondary, effects of glucocorticoids are to induce the synthesis of transaminases concerned in the formation of keto acid precursors from amino acids and to stimulate the synthesis of gluconeogenic enzymes concerned in the synthesis of glucose from the keto acids. Insulin would seem to have an opposite regulatory effect on liver metabolism in that it may induce the synthesis of glycolytic enzymes and possibly suppress certain gluconeogenic enzymes.

The antianabolic action of glucocorticoids on protein, if carried to excess, could lead to muscle wasting, reabsorption of bone matrix along with calcium, possible increased blood sugar, and increased glycogen deposition in the liver. Some of the increased glucose from noncarbohydrate sources may be diverted to fat, especially leading to a centripetal deposition of fat. A normal physiologic role of the glucocorticoids, however, is to provide glucose intermediates from amino acids derived from protein during periods of starvation or when dietary intake of carbohydrate is insufficient.

Other important functions of the glucocorticoids are their antiallergic and antiinflammatory actions. Glucocorticoids can cause an initial lysis of the lymph nodes with increased release of antibodies. There is an eventual decreased production of antibodies. The glucocorticoid hormones decrease the cellular response to noxious or infectious agents by decreasing the accumulation of neutrophils and lymphocytes. They decrease the exudative inflammatory response. By decreasing the formation of histamine and histamine-like substances in cells, they reduce the allergic response.

Thus, glucocorticoids by inhibiting protein synthesis in muscle increase the release of amino acids for conversion to glucose in the liver. Glucocorticoids also depress metabolic processes in lymphoid and adipose tissues. All of these functions of the glucocorticoids will be considered later in some detail insofar as the mechanism of action is known or postulated.

First we will examine the effect of glucocorticoids on gluconeogenesis in the liver and, at the same time, some aspects of the regulatory effect of other hormones on liver metabolism. The liver is a principal site of homeostasis for glucose. It stores excess glucose as glycogen at times when the carbohydrate intake exceeds the rate of utilization of glucose. On the other hand, the liver can convert amino acids and amino acid intermediates from muscle and other tissues to carbohydrate intermediates. A great deal of lactate is generated in muscle during intense exercise. The blood lactate can rise to as high as 10 mM. The liver can convert this lactate to pyruvate and, through gluconeogenic pathways, back to glucose. Thus, the liver has the major function of providing glucose for metabolism by other tissues that depend either solely or to a large extent on it.

Red blood cells derive their energy by glycolysis, which is the metabolism of glucose to pyruvate or lactate. The central nervous system cannot readily oxidize fatty acids and generates energy by glycolysis and the further oxidation of pyruvate through the citric acid cycle. Skeletal muscle, and especially heart muscle, can efficiently oxidize fatty acids for energy production, in addition to having an ability to oxidize glucose. The oxidation of fatty acids is insufficient to provide the extra energy needed for sudden intense muscular activity. This is provided by an increased oxidation of glucose. Much of this is metabolized by the muscle only as far as pyruvate. Pyruvate accumulates and is reduced to lactate, reoxidizing NADH. Tissues such as red cells, central nervous system, and muscle are not able to synthesize glucose from pyruvate or lactate and are dependent upon receiving glucose either in the diet or from the liver by gluconeogenesis.

GLYCOLYSIS AND GLUCONEOGENESIS

Decrease in Blood Sugar

The acute effects of a decrease in blood sugar and the hormone adaptations that can occur are outlined in Figure 1. The acute responses to a drop in the level of the blood glucose can be summarized as follows. When blood glucose drops, glucagon is released from the alpha cells of the pancreas, and epinephrine is released from the adrenal medulla. Of the two hormones, glucagon is the major factor in mediating glucose release from the liver. The reason this is so is that the level of epinephrine needed to stimulate the breakdown of glycogen to glucose is higher than that found physiologically in normal circumstances.

Glucagon, through the same series of enzyme reactions described below for epinephrine, indirectly activates the enzyme phosphorylase *a* in the liver, leading to the breakdown of glycogen to glucose with the release of glucose to contribute to blood sugar homeostasis. Glucagon also activates liver lipase for an increased breakdown of liver lipid with a release of free fatty acids and glycerol.

Epinephrine has several regulatory effects. By a series of reactions, it leads to an increase in the liver enzyme, phosphorylase *a*, which catalyzes glycogen breakdown and again contributes glucose for as long as the stores of glycogen remain. Epinephrine does this, according to Sutherland and co-workers, by stimulating the enzyme adenyl cyclase, which converts adenosine triphosphate to the cyclic adenylic acid, adenosine 3′,5′-monophosphate (3′,5′-AMP). This compound in turn stimulates phosphorylase kinase which, in the presence of ATP, converts the inactive enzyme phosphorylase *b* to the active phosphorylase *a*. The latter enzyme degrades glycogen to glucose-1-phosphate. These reactions are shown in Figure 2. Epinephrine also stimulates lipase in the adipose tissue, releasing free fatty acid and glycerol. Free fatty acid inhibits the activity of key glycolytic enzymes in the liver. Epinephrine also has an effect in stimulating the release of lactate from muscle, again providing some precursors for gluconeogenesis.

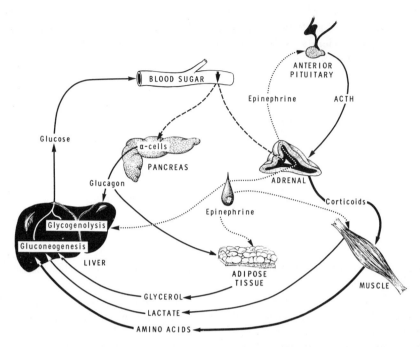

Fig. 1. Changes induced after a decrease in blood sugar. When blood sugar drops, glucagon is released from the pancreas and epinephrine from the adrenal medulla. These two hormones have a similar effect in stimulating glycogen breakdown (glycogenolysis). Both hormones also stimulate lipase in adipose tissue, resulting in the release of fatty acids and glycerol. Fatty acids inhibit key glycolytic enzymes in the liver and thus the metabolism of glucose by glycolysis. Epinephrine also stimulates the release of lactate from muscle. Epinephrine triggers the release of ACTH from the anterior pituitary, and increased ACTH stimulates the synthesis of corticoids from the adrenal cortex. Glucocorticoids inhibit protein synthesis in muscle and other tissues, increasing the release of amino acids to the liver. The increased amino acids, after transamination and the formation of keto acids, provide substrates to gluconeogenic pathways in the liver for the synthesis of glucose. (Drawn from Weber. *In* McKerns, ed. *Functions of the Adrenal Cortex.* Appleton-Century-Crofts, 1968, Vol. 2.)

In addition, epinephrine is apparently a mediator in stimulating the release of ACTH from the anterior pituitary in response to a decrease in blood glucose. Whether epinephrine is the prime or only mediator triggered by low blood glucose for the release of ACTH is uncertain. In any case, the increased ACTH stimulates the adrenal cortex for an increased production of corticoids. The glucocorticoids inhibit protein synthesis, and normal protein catabolism leads to an increased release of free amino acids from muscle and other tissues. If fasting or a high-protein, low-carbohydrate diet continues, the stimulatory effect of epinephrine on glycogen breakdown could deplete the stores of liver glycogen. The supply of glycerol from adipose tissue would be insufficient to provide carbohydrate precursor. Thus, inhibition of peripheral protein synthesis by glucocorticoids to provide amino acids would become the principal source of

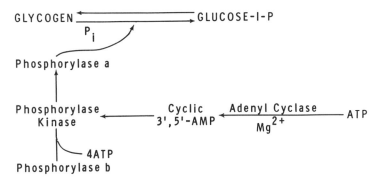

Fig. 2. The regulation of glycogen breakdown in the liver by certain hormones is at the level of adenyl cyclase. Glucagon and catecholamines such as epinephrine stimulate adenyl cyclase, which converts adenosine triphosphate (ATP) to cyclic $3',5'$-AMP. Cyclic $3',5'$-AMP stimulates phosphorylase kinase, which forms phosphorylase *a* from the inactive precursor. Phosphorylase *a* degrades glycogen to glucose-1-phosphate. Glucose-1-P is rapidly converted to glucose-6-phosphate by phosphoglucomutase. Insulin inhibits adenyl cyclase or stimulates phosphodiesterase, which converts cyclic $3',5'$-AMP to the inactive $5'$-AMP. Epinephrine also stimulates adenyl cyclase in adipose tissue. The increase in cyclic $3',5'$-AMP stimulates lipid breakdown to fatty acids, as well as the degradation of glycogen.

gluconeogenic precursors for conversion by the liver to glucose. Glucocorticoids also rapidly induce the synthesis of certain hepatic gluconeogenic enzymes and transaminases, as will be explained later.

Increase in Blood Sugar

An opposite chain of events occurs when blood sugar rises after ingestion of a meal containing carbohydrates. An elevated blood sugar level stimulates the release of insulin from the β cells of the pancreas. Insulin lowers the level of blood glucose by increasing the availability of glucose to the cell for oxidation or for storage as glycogen or lipid. The exact mechanisms involved are not yet known. Over the years, numerous possibilities have been suggested. According to Jefferson and associates, insulin directly suppresses glucose production by the liver, possibly because insulin can inhibit adenyl cyclase and lower the level of cyclic $3',5'$-AMP. This would be antagonistic to the action of glucagon or epinephrine on glycogen breakdown. These authors suggest that an important regulatory effect on glucose output from glycogen by the liver is achieved by the balance between glucagon and epinephrine in stimulating the synthesis of cyclic AMP and the effect of insulin in inhibiting the synthesis of cyclic AMP. The chain of events in the action of cyclic AMP was discussed earlier.

There is still controversy as to whether insulin stimulates the conversion of glucose to glucose-6-phosphate by the activation of glucokinase. The effect of this would be to make glucose-6-phosphate available for oxidation by glycolysis, by the pentose phosphate pathway or other metabolic processes, leading to energy production. Or if glucose-6-phosphate is in excess for the metabolic requirements of the cell, it could be stored as glycogen or converted to fatty acids and stored as lipid. On the other hand, the primary effect of insulin may be to stimulate the transport of glucose into cells and in this manner make glucose available for metabolic processes. The essence of the controversy would be whether glucose requires a transport mechanism or whether it is freely diffusable into cells. If glucose is freely available to the cell, then it could be assumed that the effect of insulin is on some rate-limiting enzyme concerned in the metabolism of glucose.

Glucose Homeostasis

The metabolism of glucose to pyruvic acid by glycolysis and the transamination of amino acids to keto acids such as pyruvic or oxalacetic, and their metabolism by gluconeogenesis, are compared in Figure 3. Glucose is metabolized to pyruvate because of the unidirectional enzymes glucokinase, phosphofructokinase, and pyruvate kinase. The direction of gluconeogenesis is regulated by another group of unidirectional enzymes, indicated in Figure 3 by the heavy arrows. By transaminations some amino acids yield pyruvate, which is converted by pyruvate carboxylase to oxalacetate. Other amino acids yield oxalacetate, which can be metabolized by phosphoenolpyruvate carboxykinase to phosphoenolpyruvate (PEP). This compound is directed to glucose by two other gluconeogenic enzymes, fructose-1,6-diphosphatase and glucose-6-phosphatase. Bidirectional enzymes function with either pathway depending on substrate concentrations, and are illustrated by the two-way arrows. All of these reactions will be considered in detail.

Glucocorticoids and Transamination

As stated earlier, an acute effect of the glucocorticoids is to inhibit protein synthesis in muscle and certain tissues. With decreased protein synthesis, degradation of protein releases amino acids into the plasma. This provides amino acids that are converted by liver transaminases to pyruvate or oxalacetate, or to dicarboxylic acids that can be metabolized by the citric acid cycle to oxalacetate. Excess protein intake also provides amino acids. These metabolites derived from amino acids by transamination can be converted to phosphoenolpyruvate, as we shall see later, and enter the pathways of synthesis to glucose. Metabolism of glucose by skeletal muscle also provides pyruvate, or lactate that can be oxidized to pyruvate by lactic dehydrogenase in the presence of NAD^+. Some mechanisms of transamination of certain amino acids to gluconeogenic substrates are illustrated as follows.

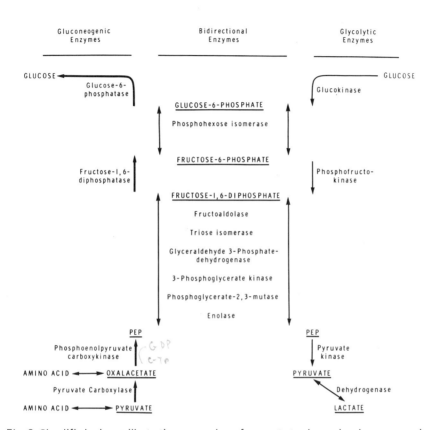

Fig. 3. Simplified scheme illustrating conversion of pyruvate to glucose by gluconeogenesis, and glucose to pyruvate by glycolysis in the liver. Unidirectional enzymes in gluconeogesis are pyruvate carboxylase, phosphoenolpyruvate carboxykinase, fructose-1,6-diphosphatase and glucose-6-phosphatase. Unidirectional enzymes in glycolysis are glucokinase, phosphofructokinase, and pyruvate kinase. Other enzymes connecting these pathways work in either direction, depending on substrate concentrations and are called bidirectional. An additional bifunctional enzyme is phosphoglucomutase which interconverts glucose-6-phosphate and glucose-1-phosphate. Glucose-1-phosphate may be converted to glycogen or derived from glycogen relative to glucose-6-phosphate concentration.

When blood sugar is low, glucocorticoids suppress protein synthesis in muscle and other tissues. Increased amino acids are available to the liver for metabolism and transamination to keto acids, such as pyruvate and oxalacetate. The keto acids are converted to glucose, much of which is released from the liver as a metabolite for muscle, brain, red cells, and other tissues, which are dependent on glucose as an energy source.

When blood glucose is high after ingestion of carbohydrate, insulin is released, which stimulates the metabolism of glucose to pyruvate and its metabolism by the citric acid cycle as an energy source for liver function. Excess glucose is stored as glycogen, or pyruvate can form acetyl-CoA used in fatty acid synthesis. In addition, pyruvate or keto acids arising from pyruvate in the citric acid cycle can be transaminated to amino acids.

$$
\begin{array}{cc}
\text{COO}^- & \\
| & \\
\text{C=O} & \\
| & \text{COO}^- \\
\text{CH}_2 & | \\
| & \overset{+}{\text{H}_3}\text{N–CH} \\
\text{CH}_2 & | \\
| & \text{R} \\
\text{COO}^- &
\end{array}
\qquad
\begin{array}{cc}
\text{COO}^- & \\
| & \\
\overset{+}{\text{H}_3}\text{N–CH} & \\
| & \text{COO}^- \\
\text{CH}_2 & | \\
| & \text{C=O} \\
\text{CH}_2 & | \\
| & \text{R} \\
\text{COO}^- &
\end{array}
$$

α-KETOGLUTARIC ACID + AMINO ACID ⟷ GLUTAMIC ACID + α-KETO ACID

Fig. 4. General mechanism of transamination. α-Ketoglutarate is the common acceptor of -NH$_3$$^+$ from amino acids. Pyridoxal phosphate is a common cofactor of transaminase reactions.

A general route of transamination is by transfer of the -NH$_3^+$ of the amino acid to α-ketoglutarate by liver transaminases specific for certain amino acids. This yields a keto acid and glutamic acid as shown in Figure 4.

Liver mitochondria have a high activity of glutamic acid dehydrogenase so that α-ketoglutaric acid can be regenerated:

$$\text{glutamic acid} + \text{NAD}^+ + \text{H}_2\text{O} \longleftrightarrow \text{α-ketoglutaric acid} + \text{NADH} + \text{NH}_4^+$$

The reaction goes to the right when glutamic acid is in excess. The NADH may be oxidized by the mitochondrial electron transport system. The NH$_4^+$ can enter the urea cycle of the liver, where the ammonia can be excreted as urea. These two reactions, with the NH$_4^+$ coupled to the urea cycle, can constitute a cyclic system for removing -NH$_3^+$ from amino acids with a net yield of keto acids as glucose precursors. α-Ketoglutarate is the common acceptor of -NH$_3^+$ in the transamination reactions. Of course, the reverse reactions can occur—namely, the amination of keto acids by transamination from glutamate. This is important in the synthesis of amino acids (so called nonessential) from keto acids derived from glucose when glucose is in excess and dietary intake of protein is limited. The amination of keto acids by transamination from glutamate is an essential reaction in the synthesis of urea, as discussed later.

Thus amino acids such as alanine can be deaminated to yield the keto acid pyruvate, as shown in Figure 5.

Pyridoxal phosphate is a prosthetic group or working part of these transaminase enzymes in that it is involved in the transfer of ammonia. Another example is the transamination of aspartate, which can be converted by glutamate-oxalacetate transaminase directly to oxalacetate as shown in Figure 6.

Amino acids such as histidine and proline can be converted to glutamate, and glutamate itself can enter the citric acid cycle by conversion to α-ketoglutarate. The glucocorticoids, in addition to increasing the catabolism of

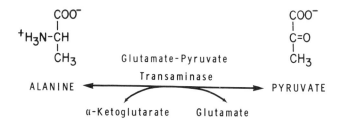

Fig. 5. The glutamate-pyruvate transaminase reaction. With α-ketoglutarate as the acceptor of $-NH_3^+$ from alanine, pyruvate can be formed. The reverse reaction can be used for the synthesis of alanine.

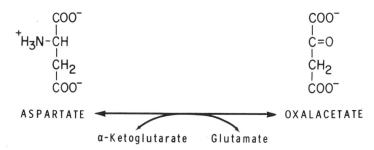

Fig. 6. The glutamate-oxalacetate transaminase reaction. Oxalacetate can be formed from aspartate with α-ketoglutarate as the acceptor of $-NH_3^+$ from aspartate. When oxalacetate is in excess, the reverse reaction can occur.

protein to amino acids, also induce an early increase in the activity of liver transaminases.

So amino acids by various reactions, some of which are illustrated above, yield either pyruvate, oxalacetate, α-ketoglutarate, or other keto acids. Pyruvate, α-ketoglutarate, and other keto acids can be metabolized to oxalacetate. Excess oxalacetate not metabolized by the mitochondria for the synthesis of ATP is available for synthesis to glucose by gluconeogenesis. This occurs via the transformation of oxalacetate to phosphoenolpyruvate.

Metabolism of Keto Acids

Pyruvate and oxalacetate derived from the amino acids enter gluconeogenic pathways in the liver by conversion to phosphoenolpyruvate (PEP), as shown in Figure 7. The first reaction requires adenosine triphosphate (ATP) as an energy source, and the second reaction requires guanosine triphosphate (GTP). Thus, pyruvate formed by transamination from amino acids such as

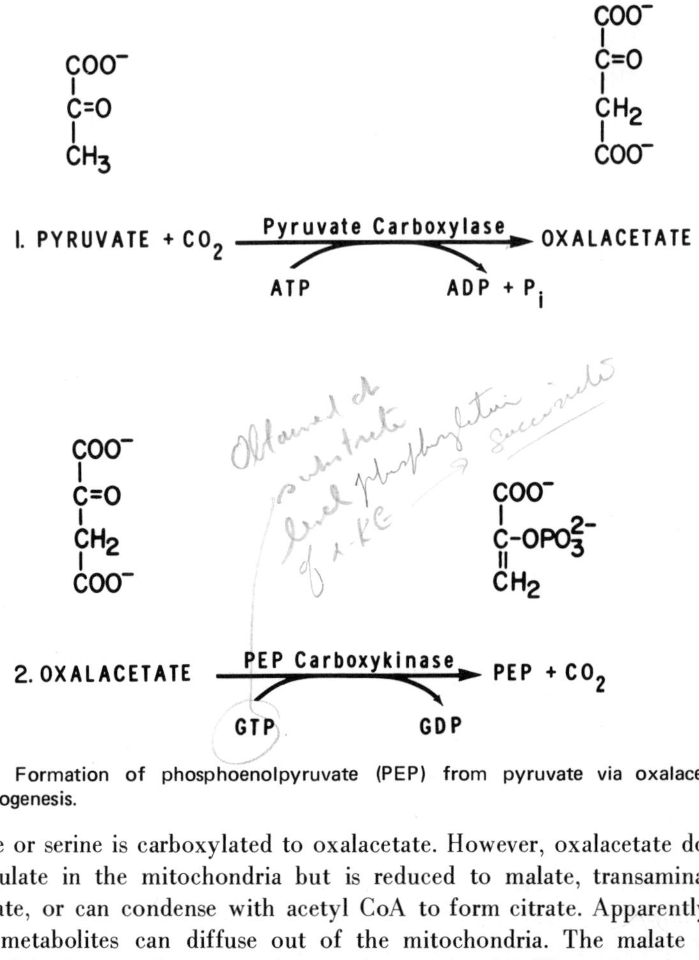

$$
\begin{array}{c}
COO^- \\
| \\
C=O \\
| \\
CH_3
\end{array}
\qquad\qquad
\begin{array}{c}
COO^- \\
| \\
C=O \\
| \\
CH_2 \\
| \\
COO^-
\end{array}
$$

1. PYRUVATE + CO_2 $\xrightarrow[\text{ATP} \quad\quad \text{ADP} + P_i]{\text{Pyruvate Carboxylase}}$ OXALACETATE

$$
\begin{array}{c}
COO^- \\
| \\
C=O \\
| \\
CH_2 \\
| \\
COO^-
\end{array}
\qquad\qquad
\begin{array}{c}
COO^- \\
| \\
C-OPO_3^{2-} \\
\| \\
CH_2
\end{array}
$$

2. OXALACETATE $\xrightarrow[\text{GTP} \quad\quad\quad \text{GDP}]{\text{PEP Carboxykinase}}$ PEP + CO_2

(handwritten annotation: Obtained at substrate level phosphorylation like of α-KG → succinate)

Fig. 7. Formation of phosphoenolpyruvate (PEP) from pyruvate via oxalacetate in gluconeogenesis.

alanine or serine is carboxylated to oxalacetate. However, oxalacetate does not accumulate in the mitochondria but is reduced to malate, transaminated to aspartate, or can condense with acetyl CoA to form citrate. Apparently these three metabolites can diffuse out of the mitochondria. The malate can be oxidized in the cytoplasm to oxalacetate by reaction 4 in Figure 8, and aspartate transaminated to oxalacetate. Oxalacetate, now outside the mitochondria, is available for conversion to phosphoenolpyruvate.

This mitochondrial "shuttle" of substrates such as malate and aspartate has been postulated by Lardy and co-workers for the rat or other species where PEP carboxykinase is found in the cytoplasm. In the rabbit, PEP carboxykinase is located in the mitochondria, and in the guinea pig is found in both the mitochondria and cytoplasm. Citrate cleavage back to oxalacetate and acetyl-CoA is apparently not an induced mechanism in gluconeogenesis.

(handwritten margin note: Loca of PEP kinase)

Haslam and Krebs have studied the permeability of rat liver, kidney, and heart mitochondria to oxalacetate and malate. The maximal translocation of oxalacetate requires an energy source such as ATP. The permeability of

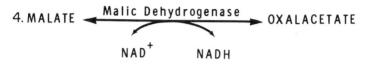

3. PYRUVATE $+ CO_2$ $\xleftarrow{\text{Malic Enzyme}}\rightarrow$ MALATE

NADPH   NADP$^+$

4. MALATE $\xleftarrow{\text{Malic Dehydrogenase}}\rightarrow$ OXALACETATE

NAD$^+$ NADH

Fig. 8. Malic enzyme and malic dehydrogenase enzyme reactions. The conversion of pyruvate to malate is apparently less important in gluconeogenesis than pyruvate carboxylase, shown in Figure 7. However, oxalacetate is reduced to malate in the mitochondria by mitochondrial malic dehydrogenase. Malate diffusing out of the mitochondria is oxidized back to oxalacetate by malic dehydrogenase outside the mitochondria. Thus reducing equivalents are removed from mitochondrial metabolism, and NADH is provided for gluconeogenesis for the conversion of 1,3-diphosphoglycerate to glyceraldehyde-3-phosphate, shown in Figure 11. Oxalacetate is also provided for the extramitochondrial conversion to PEP. In summary, excess oxalacetate in the mitochondria is reduced to malate, which, on diffusing out, is oxidized by a cytoplasmic malic dehydrogenase which acts in the direction malate to oxalacetate.

mitochondria to oxalacetate is restricted without such energy. However, Haslam and Krebs have provided further evidence that malate is an important carrier of hydrogen between mitochondria and cytoplasm. In the metabolism of glucose by glycolysis, each molecule yields two molecules of pyruvate and of NADH. Pyruvate can form oxalacetate by the pyruvate carboxylase reaction. Oxalacetate can be reduced to malate by an NAD$^+$-malic dehydrogenase. Malate enters the mitochondria, and malate dehydrogenase inside provides oxalacetate and reduces NAD$^+$. In this way, malate could provide both oxalacetate and a reducing equivalent for mitochondrial metabolism. During the early steps of gluconeogenesis, hydrogen equivalents and oxalacetate can be transferred out of the mitochondria in the form of malate by the reverse of the processes described above.

The major conversion of pyruvate to oxalacetate and thence to PEP in the liver during gluconeogenesis could go via the reactions discussed above rather than through an NADP$^+$-malic enzyme linked to malic dehydrogenase to form oxalacetate, as illustrated in reactions 3 and 4 in Figure 8. The NADP$^+$-malate enzymes may not be important in gluconeogenesis, but may well have an important function in capturing extramitochondrial NADPH required in steroid hydroxylations in mitochondria of the adrenal cortex and other endocrine tissues. This is discussed in the section on electron flow in the adrenal cortex.

Reaction 4 in Figure 8 (malate to oxalacetate), when it occurs outside the mitochondria, is useful in providing NADH required during gluconeogenesis for the conversion of 1,3-diphosphoglycerate to D-glyceraldehyde-3-phosphate. This reaction is illustrated later under bifunctional enzymes. Thus, malate of mitochondrial origin derived from oxalacetate could provide reducing equivalents in the cytoplasm, as well as oxalacetate.

In summary, one route of metabolism of pyruvate is its carboxylation to oxalacetate in the mitochondria, reduction to malate by NADH-malate dehydrogenase, with diffusion of malate out of the mitochondria. Malate is then oxidized to oxalacetate by extramitochondrial NAD^+-malic dehydrogenase, with NAD^+ reduced to NADH. Another possible route would be the intramitochondrial conversion of oxalacetate to aspartate and diffusion of aspartate out of the mitochondria. Aspartate then could be transaminated back to oxalacetate, or converted to malate through fumarate and the urea cycle.

In the later step of glycolysis, the conversion of phosphoenolpyruvate occurs by the pyruvate kinase reaction and yields ATP as shown in Figure 9. The reverse of this reaction does not occur under physiologic conditions.

In Figure 10 the formation of pyruvate from phosphoenolpyruvate during glycolysis is contrasted with the formation of phosphoenolpyruvate from pyruvate via oxalacetate during gluconeogenesis. This entry of gluconeogenic amino acids into gluconeogenic pathways, via pyruvate, oxalacetate, succinyl-CoA, or α-ketoglutarate, is also indicated by arrows. The metabolism of these compounds to oxalacetate and thus to PEP is shown. It was mentioned that α-ketoglutarate was the common acceptor of $-NH_3^+$ in the transamination of amino acids to keto acids. The glutamate so formed can contribute $-NH_3^+$ to the urea cycle by two reactions. Ammonia from the glutamate dehydrogenase reaction enters the urea cycle via the formation of carbamyl phosphate. Ammonia can also come from glutamate by its transformation to a semialdehyde and subsequent transamination, regenerating α-ketoglutarate.

Bifunctional Enzymes

As is apparent from the foregoing, gluconeogenesis is not just the reverse of glycolysis. In other words, there are certain unique enzymes for each process. However, some enzymes are shared by both glycolysis and glyconeogenesis and are called by Weber "bifunctional enzymes." They are considered to be present in excess and thus are not rate limiting. They work in either direction depending on the substrate concentration. With the possible exception of lactic dehydrogenase, they are apparently not activated by, nor is their synthesis induced by,

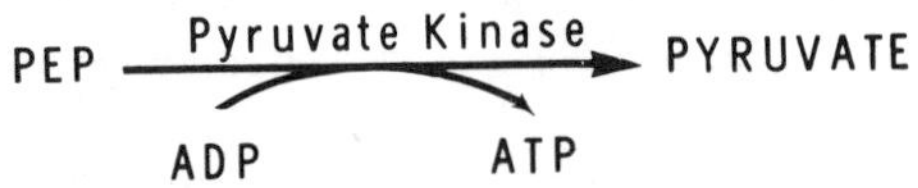

PEP $\xrightarrow{\text{Pyruvate Kinase}}$ PYRUVATE

ADP   ATP

Fig. 9. The conversion of phosphoenolpyruvate (PEP) to pyruvate, with the formation of ATP, is the final, irreversible step of glycolysis under physiologic conditions.

hormones. These enzymes between glucose and lactate are phosphoglucomutase, phosphohexoseisomerase, fructoaldolase, trioseisomerase, glyceraldehyde-3-phosphate dehydrogenase, 3-phosphoglycerate kinase, phosphoglycerate-2, 3-mutase, enolase, and lactate dehydrogenase. They are indicated in the summary Figure 14 by the two-way arrows. The specific two-way reactions of the bifunctional enzymes are illustrated in Figure 11, except for phosphoglucomutase and phosphohexoseisomerase (phosphoglucoisomerase), which are shown in Figure 13, and lactate dehydrogenase, shown in Figure 12.

Key Gluconeogenic Enzymes

There are four key unidirectional enzymes in gluconeogenesis which govern the rate of glucose synthesis from pyruvate; the important control functions of these enzymes were indicated by Krebs and subsequently have been confirmed extensively. They are pyruvate carboxylase and phosphoenolpyruvate carboxykinase, mentioned previously as enzymes linking pyruvate and oxalacetate to phosphoenolpyruvate in the glyconeogenic path to glucose; fructose-1, 6-diphosphatase, which converts fructose-1,6-diphosphate to fructose-6-phosphate; and glucose-6-phosphatase, which converts glucose-6-phosphate to glucose for release from the liver.

The reactions of the two latter enzymes are illustrated in Figure 13 along with the two opposing glycolytic enzymes. Phosphohexoseisomerase and phosphoglucomutase are bifunctional enzymes. Metabolism of fructose-1,6-diphosphate to phosphoenolpyruvate is by bifunctional enzymes, for which reactions are given in Figure 11.

When blood glucose drops and the supply of glucose for brain, muscle, and other tissues becomes limited, protein synthesis is inhibited and amino acids are converted to pyruvate and oxalacetate, or decarboxylic acids for conversion to oxalacetate in the mitochondrial citric acid cycle. These enzymatic processes have been described, as well as the inhibitory effect of glucocorticoids on protein synthesis. The substrates derived from amino acids flow through the gluconeogenic enzymes and the bifunctional enzymes to yield glucose. One effect of glucocorticoids is, then, to stimulate amino acid catabolism from tissue or ingested protein and thus to provide substrates for glucose synthesis. The glucocorticoids also have an effect in inducing the synthesis of the key gluconeogenic enzymes relative to the necessity for gluconeogenesis. An increased activity of transaminase enzymes is also apparent in the liver after the administration of glutocorticoids to animals. For example, tyrosine-ketoglutarate transaminase has been studied in rat liver as a model enzyme that is easily induced after cortisol administration. Enzymes such as phosphoenolpyruvate carboxykinase are fairly rapidly induced in the liver by the administration of hydrocortisone to the rat, reaching a maximum activity in about four hours. However, the primary effect of glucocorticoids may be to inhibit protein

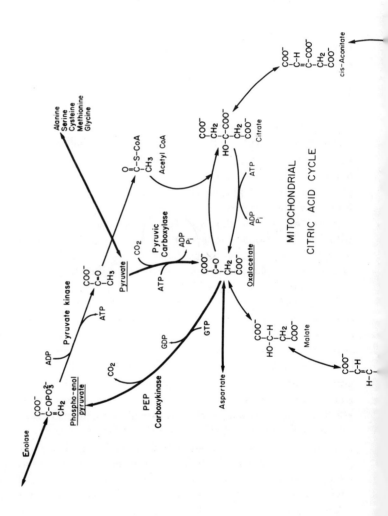

44

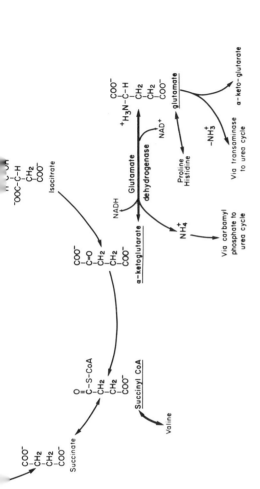

Fig. 10. This figure summarizes the reactions of the liver, discussed so far, in transamination, the formation of pyruvate from phosphoenolpyruvate in glycolysis, and the formation of phosphoenolpyruvate from oxalacetate in gluconeogenesis. During gluconeogenesis, excess oxalacetate is reduced to malate in the mitochondria by malic dehydrogenase (oxalacetate + NADH → malate + NAD^+). Malate diffuses out, and malic dehydrogenase outside the mitochondria reoxidizes malate to oxalacetate, and NAD^+ is reduced. In addition, oxalacetate is transaminated to aspartate in the mitochondria. Aspartate diffuses out and is transaminated back to oxalacetate. Thus, oxalacetate actually reformed outside the mitochondria from malate or aspartate, can enter the gluconeogenic pathway via the PEP carboxykinase reaction. Transamination and other reactions of the amino acids alanine, serine, cysteine, methionine, and glycine can yield pyruvate, glutamate can yield α-ketoglutarate, valine can give succinyl-CoA, as substrates for the citric acid cycle. Aspartate can be directly transaminated to oxalacetate. The association of glutamate dehydrogenase and the release of NH_4^+ to the urea cycle is indicated.

During glycolysis, oxalacetate mostly condenses with acetyl-CoA to form citrate, which can be metabolized by the citric acid cycle as shown. Hydrogens are captured in the reactions isocitrate to α-ketoglutarate, succinate to fumarate, and malate to oxalacetate. Mitochondrial electron transport for the synthesis of ATP from ADP, or for hydroxylation and reductive reactions, in steroid inactivation, are similar to those discussed for adrenal mitochondria.

Citrate cleavage also releases oxalacetate and acetyl-CoA outside the mitochondria. This reaction is more important in fatty acid synthesis than in gluconeogenesis.

The relative rates of these various reactions depend on the needs of the cell, the availability of substrates from various sources, and the induction or suppression of various extramitochondrial enzymes, as explained in the text and in Figure 14.

45

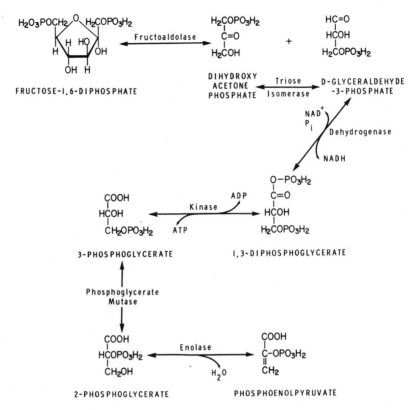

Fig. 11. Bifunctional enzymes in the liver that work with glycolytic enzymes or gluconeogenic enzymes, depending on substrate concentrations. These are phosphoglu-comutase and phosphohexoseisomerase shown in Figure 13, along with fructoaldolase, trioseisomerase, D-glyceraldehyde-3-phosphate dehydrogenase, 1,3-diphosphoglycerate kinase, 3-phosphoglycerate mutase, enolase, and lactate dehydrogenase (Figure 12).

Fig. 12. Reactions of the lactate dehydrogenase enzyme.

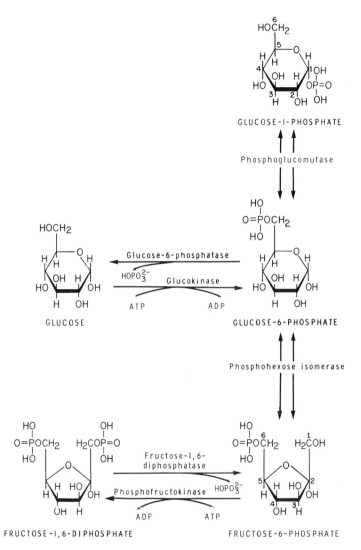

Fig. 13. The four key gluconeogenic enzymes are pyruvate carboxylase and phosphoenol-pyruvate carboxykinase, shown in Figure 7, along with fructose-1,6-diphosphatase and glucose-6-phosphatase, shown above. Also illustrated above are two of the three key glycolytic enzymes, glucokinase and phosphofructokinase, and two bifunctional enzymes, phosphoglucomutase and phosphoglucoisomerase (phosphohexoseisomerase). The third key glycolytic enzyme is pyruvic kinase, shown in Figure 9.

synthesis in tissues other than the liver rather than an induction of gluconeo-genic and transaminase enzymes of the liver. But enzyme induction is at least a secondary effect of glucocorticoids, though not necessarily a direct action of the hormones. In addition, glucocorticoids may have a suppressing effect on the synthesis or activity of the glucolytic enzymes. Again, the could be due to changes in substrate levels, rather than direct inhibitory effects of glucocorticoids.

Moreover, fatty acids have an acute effect in inhibiting glycolytic enzymes. Fatty acid oxidation in liver mitochondria also provides reducing equivalents as FADH and NADH, used in the synthesis of ATP, as well as acetyl-CoA. Thus, fatty acid oxidation would reduce the necessity for metabolism of pyruvate to acetyl-CoA and divert the metabolism of pyruvate to oxalacetate.

Weber has suggested that the four gluconeogenic enzymes are induced together, possibly by stimulating or de-repressing an "operon" on a genic unit having a DNA sequence for the synthesis of mRNA's for all four enzymes. This would be according to the "operon" concepts of Jacob and Monod. However, there is no proof for this possible hormone mechanism nor for Weber's interesting concept that all four enzymes derive from one genomic unit and are synthesized together. The idea of one genic unit for the four gluconeogenic enzymes is also difficult to reconcile with the fact that these enzymes may be found in different cellular fractions.

Key Glycolytic Enzymes

The other set of three enzymes working in a unidirectional fashion, in conjunction with the bifunctional or bidirectional enzymes, are the essential or "key" glycolytic enzymes. These are glucokinase, concerned in the phosphorylation of glucose to glucose-6-phosphate; phosphofructokinase, which utilizes ATP for the phosphorylation of fructose-6-phosphate to fructose-1,6-diphosphate (shown in Figure 13); and finally, pyruvic kinase, which generates ATP in the conversion of phosphoenolpyruvate to pyruvate. Pyruvate kinase is shown in Figure 9. Pyruvate is, then, available to mitochondrial reactions via the formation of acetyl-CoA and oxalacetate. Pyruvate can also be reduced to lactate by the lactate dehydrogenase reaction and NADH (Fig. 12).

Weber suggests that the three key glycolytic enzymes are induced together on a single genic unit. In this case the inducer could be insulin, released from the β cells of the pancreas when blood sugar is elevated. Or increased levels of glycolytic substrates derived from glucose could be the inducers of glycolytic enzymes. By analogy to the gluconeogenic enzymes, glucocorticoids probably would act indirectly, as suppressors to the glycolytic enzymes. Thus, there would be a reciprocal relation between glycolytic and glucneogenic enzymes, with induction and suppression by insulin and glucocorticoids as described. However, the reciprocal behavior of all key enzymes of each pathway may not always occur.

Takeda and associates suggest from their data that only glucokinase of the key glycolytic enzymes may be regulated by insulin and that the activity of pyruvate kinase may be regulated by the flow of metabolites through the glycolytic pathway. Ray and Ray, Foster, and Lardy feel that the primary effect of glucocorticoids is not on enzyme induction in gluconeogenesis but is obviously important for the maximum expression of the effect on carbohydrate systhesis. However, they suggest that enzyme induction is a secondary occurrence derived from a primary effect of glucocorticoids in providing metabolites from amino acids for the enzymes of gluconeogeniesis. Increased concentrations of gluconeogenic substrates could de-repress the DNA-control systems concerned in the synthesis of these enzymes. So there are some details to be resolved. Nevertheless, the general principal of two pathways, one for the synthesis of glucose from amino acids or other intermediates, and one for the metabolism of glucose to pyruvate with each pathway sharing bidirectional enzymes, is well established.

Pathways of Substrate Metabolism in Gluconeogenesis

A scheme illustrating the flow of metabolites through the two pathways is outlined in Figure 14. The direction of metabolism of pyruvate to oxalacetate to glucose by gluconeogenesis is illustrated by heavy arrows.

In summary then, the synthesis of glucose from lactate, pyruvate, and certain amino acids by gluconeogenesis differs from the direct reversal of glycolysis at certain key enzymatic steps. Thermodynamically, the glycolytic enzymes—glucokinase, phosphofructokinase, and pyruvate kinase—are essentially irreversible under physiologic conditions. These reactions are circumvented by glucose-6-phosphatase, fructose-1,6-diphosphatase, and the dicarboxylic acid shuttle. This last pathway involves the carboxylation of pyruvate to oxalacetate by pyruvate carboxylase and the phosphorylative decarboxylation of oxalacetate to phosphoenolpyruvate (PEP) by phosphoenolpyruvate carboxykinase. As explained in this chapter, the induction or suppression of these enzymes by hormones, whether as a primary or secondary effect, regulates glucose oxidation or glucose synthesis. The dietary intake of glucose is a major factor in initiating the secretion of the hormones involved.

Of further interest is the fact that the fetal animal does not synthesize glucose or glycogen until birth and is dependent upon maternal glucose during fetal life. After full-term birth, gluconeogenesis begins and is characterized at least in part by a marked increase in PEP carboxykinase.

The liver of the diabetic animal has elevated levels of the gluconeogenic enzymes—glucose-6-phosphatase, fructose-1,6-diphosphatase, phosphoenolpyruvate carboxykinase, and pyruvate carboxylase. In the absence of insulin to stimulate the transport of glucose into the cell, a higher concentration of blood glucose is required as a compensation. Increased gluconeogenesis contributes to the increased level of glucose. The elevated levels of the gluconeogenic enzymes reflect the needs for increased blood concentrations of glucose. The administration of insulin suppresses these enzymes and elevates the glycolytic enzymes, possibly by increasing the level of glycolytic substrates rather than acting directly.

Gluconeogenesis also occurs in the kidney cortex. Slices of kidney cortex have been found by Krebs to be especially suitable for studying quantitative aspects of gluconeogenesis. Unlike liver slices, slices of kidney cortex are more stable, have a low level of preformed carbohydrate since they synthesize little glycogen, and also metabolize little of the glucose formed.

Not considered in this chapter is the pentose phosphate pathway for the metabolism of glucose-6-phosphate. In the liver this pathway accounts for about

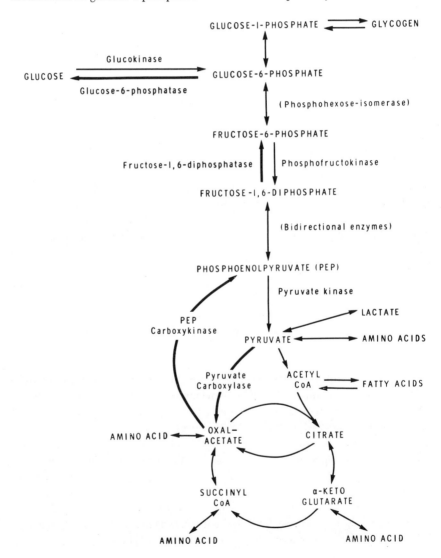

30 percent of the glucose oxidized. A principal function of the pathway is apparently to provide reducing equivalents as NADPH for fatty acid synthesis and for steroid inactivation and drug detoxification in the liver. Steroid inactivation by the liver and kidney is discussed in Chapter 8, on steroid catabolism. Fatty acid synthesis is discussed in Chapter 9, and the pentose phosphate pathway is described in detail in Chapter 2.

ADRENAL GLUCOCORTICOID HORMONES AND THE IMMUNE RESPONSE

Glucocorticoids have a number of suppressive effects on lymphatic tissues, on their ability to produce lymphocytes and antibodies, and thus on the immune response to antigen. Glucocorticoids also have an inhibitory effect on capillary dilation and leakage caused by histamine and like compounds, as well as on the histamine effect on contraction of smooth muscle. A tissue reaction to histamine is part of the inflammatory and allergic response. The response can be local, as

---

Fig. 14. Flow of metabolites in gluconeogenesis and glycolysis in the liver. This figure can also be used in conjunction with Figure 10, where certain reactions are given in more detail, such as the derivation of oxalacetate. In gluconeogenesis, amino acids can be converted to pyruvate, α-ketoglutarate, succinyl-CoA or oxalacetate outside the mitochondria, as explained in the text and under Figure 10. As explained previously, when blood sugar falls, increased breakdown of neutral lipid to fatty acid and glycerol occurs. Increased oxidation of fatty acid by the mitochondria provides reducing equivalents for ATP synthesis and supplies acetyl-CoA. Increased levels of acetyl-CoA activate pyruvate carboxylase and stimulate the synthesis of oxalacetate from pyruvate. This allows a diversion of pyruvate derived from amino acids to the pyruvate carboxylase reaction to produce excess oxalacetate. Fatty acids also inhibit the glycolytic enzymes. These acute effects probably precede the induction of gluconeogenic enzymes. PEP carboxykinase forms PEP from oxalacetate, which is converted by a series of bifunctional enzymes to fructose-1,6-diphosphate. Fructose-1,6-diphosphatase converts this latter compound to fructose-6-phosphate, which is converted to glucose-6-phosphate by phosphoglucoisomerase. Glucose-6-phosphatase forms glucose for release from the liver.

In glycolysis, glucose-6-phosphate is formed by the glucokinase reaction or from the breakdown of stored glycogen. The pathway to fructose-6-phosphate, fructose-1,6-diphosphate, phosphoenolpyruvate, and pyruvate can be followed in the diagram. Pyruvate is available for metabolism by the citric acid cycle, where electrons can be captured in the electron-transport sequence for formation of ATP or for other reactions.

When pyruvate derived by glycolysis is the major energy source, it forms acetyl-CoA in the mitochondria. This condenses with oxalacetate to form citrate. The two-carbon acetyl unit is oxidized in the citric acid cycle, and oxalacetate is regenerated. When acetyl-CoA is in excess beyond what is needed in the citric acid cycle for ATP synthesis, the increasing level of acetyl-CoA stimulates pyruvate carboxylase and the formation of oxalacetate. The respiratory chain for the synthesis of ATP is inhibited when the ratio of ATP to ADP is high, and citrate, derived from the condensation of oxalacetate and acetyl-CoA, diffuses out of the mitochondria. Citrate can provide both reducing equivalents and acetyl-CoA for the synthesis of fatty acids, as explained in the Chapter 9, on lipid metabolism.

around a wound, or more general, as in allergy or anaphylaxis. Glucocorticoids have profound effects on allergic and immune responses triggered by foreign antigens such as those in pollen or bacteria, since glucorticoids suppress the formation of antibodies and reduce the response to histamine and other inflammatory agents. When given in large amounts, they suppress the natural immune response to transplants of foreign tissue.

Anaphylaxis, hypersensitivity, and allergic reaction have been considered to be due to the production of abnormal antibodies. These abnormal antibodies attach to mast cells rather than circulating in the blood where they would bind firmly to antigen. The anaphylactic or hypersensitivity reaction would seem to be characterized by the first small stimulation by antigen of abnormal antibody that attaches to the mast cell. Mast cells probably arise from some undifferentiated mesenchymal cells of the loose connective tissue. Their origin has not been definitely established, but they are believed to contain much of the histamine of the body. If there is a second exposure to the same antigen, it apparently reacts with the antibody on the mast cells and in some fashion causes the release of histamine. Histamine and similar compounds such as 5-hydroxyhistamine cause contraction of the smooth muscle but increase dilation and permeability in the microcirculation. In people suffering from asthma, which can be considered as a milder form of the anaphylactic reaction, there is contraction of smooth muscle around the tubes through which air passes to the lungs. The tubes may be so constricted that it is difficult to breathe. Capillary dilation and leakage, at least partly due to histamine, can be observed in the capillaries close to the skin in people experiencing an anaphylactic reaction. Hives is another varient of the hypersensitivity reaction. Fluid, swelling, and redness are apparent because of the capillary leakage under the skin.

Another characteristic of hypersensitivity of tissues is a possible infiltration by mononuclear cells followed by cellular necrosis. For example, it has been demonstrated experimentally that when fibroblasts are exposed to immune lymphoid cells, lymphocytes containing antibodies aggregate around the fibroblasts. Destruction of both cell types can then occur, probably owing to rupture of lysosomal membranes by the antigen-antibody reactions, with a release of proteolytic enzymes. Glucocorticoids apparently have some stabilizing effect on the lysosome membranes, thus inhibiting their rupture and release of proteolytic enzymes.

The enzymatic lysis of foreign protein is also a normal function of neutrophils, which are the most numerous of the granular leukocytes. There is an increased release of neutrophils from the bone marrow when infection is present in the body. Phagocytosis of bacteria or other foreign protein by neutrophils involves the envelopment of the protein by the neutrophil membrane and fusion with cytoplasmic granules (lysosomes) containing proteolytic enzymes. The release of the enzymes destroys both the foreign protein and the neutrophil.

Lymphocytes important in antibody production are produced in lymphatic tissue, such as that in the loose connective tissue (also called primary or malpighian nodules), lymph nodes (or glands), the spleen, and the thymus. Except for the thymus, lymphatic tissues are all exposed to lymph circulation so that they can quickly respond to any disease organism or foreign protein antigen that enters the body. Thus, the production of lymphocytes and other cells arising from them is stimulated by antigen. These cells produce the specific gamma globulin antibodies to the antigen. Antibodies combine with antigens by H-bonding or electrostatic attraction of complementary and oppositely charged groups on the amino acid residues of the polypeptides (proteins).

The antigen-antibody reaction can be explained in the following fashion. The peptide bond in the polypeptide is the result of the reaction between the carboxyl group of one amino acid and the amino group of another with the loss of H_2O. The charged groups on polypeptides are due to dicarboxylic amino acids which have a carboxyl group (-COO^-) not involved in the peptide linkage, or to amino acids such as lysine which have an extra amino group (-NH_3^+). Hydroxyl groups (-O^-) may also be involved in H-bonding or electrostatic attraction between molecules. The overall charge of the molecules also affects their association. The more oppositely charged groups involved, the stronger the attraction. These oppositely charged groups on the two polypeptide chains (antigens in one case, antibody in the other) have to be complementary to one another. That is to say, the charge sequences of the molecules have to line up so that the opposite charge groups are within 1 or 2 angstroms of one another. The simplest arrangement would be found in a linear or primary structure of a polypeptide chain. However, since the polypeptide chains of the large antibody molecules are folded in various ways to give secondary, tertiary, or possible quaternary structures, complementariness has to adapt to these configurations. Principles relating to these concepts are discussed in the chapter on genetic control of metabolism.

The thymus is not exposed to antibodies from the lymph circulation, and only those antigens carried by the blood reach it. Even these antigens are not readily transported to the site of lymphocyte production. The prime function of the thymus in prenatal and postnatal life is to produce lymphocytes that are competent to produce antibodies, but not yet "coded" to synthesize specific antibodies. Thus, these uncommitted lymphocytes migrate to other lymphatic tissues to assist in building up their population of cells, free to respond to new antigens. Also there is some humoral factor produced by the thymic epithelium which is necessary in early prenatal life to stimulate lymphatic tissue elsewhere in the body to become immunologically competent—that is, to respond to antigen.

As stated earlier, the glucocorticoids have a marked effect on the mobilization of protein from lymphoid tissue. This is probably due to an inhibition of protein synthesis at the level of the cellular pool of free amino acids. The net effect is the suppression of function of the lymphoid tissues. This effect of glucocorticoids is probably the same as their suppressive effect on protein synthesis in muscle and some other tissues, leading to an increased pool of amino acids available for metabolism to keto acids and thence to glucose in the liver. These effects of glucocorticoids on liver metabolism and glucose homeostasis have already been considered. Some ideas concerning the effects of glucocorticoids on lymphoid tissues will be developed now.

Glucocorticoid Action on Lymphocytes

As a model system to study the effects of glucocorticoids and other agents on the metabolism of lymphoid tissues, Markman, Nakagawa, and White have developed an in vitro incubation system of lymphocyte cells. Metabolic depression of DNA, RNA, and protein synthesis was observed in vitro after either in vitro or in vivo exposure to steroids. Cell suspensions of lymphocytes in culture medium were prepared from thymic or mesenteric lymph node tissue of the rat. The medium was Eagle's spinner culture medium containing Puck's balanced salt solution. This mixture contains essential amino acids, glutamine, glucose, and vitamins. These authors found, for example, that the administration of cortisol (17α-hydroxycorticosterone) one or three hours prior to sacrifice of the rat decreased the in vitro incorporation of H^3-uridine into RNA, and H^3-deoxycytidine into nucleic acids, and C^{14}-leucine and C^{14}-glycine into protein. It was also found that the in vivo administration of cortisol as early as forty minutes prior to incubation of thymic cells in vitro significantly decreased H^3-uridine incorporation into RNA. The thymic nuclei also showed a decreased activity of RNA polymerase. Similar inhibitions of DNA, RNA, and protein were observed when cortisol at 10^{-6} M was incubated with thymocyte suspensions in vitro. Glucose or some other energy source was found necessary for an inhibitory effect of cortisol, especially on the inhibition of uridine incorporation into RNA. Other experiments demonstrated an inhibitory effect on transport into thymocytes. Thus, the inhibitory effects of glucocorticoids appear to be at two loci: a transport site regulating the transfer of nucleic acid and protein precursors into the thymocytes, and an intracellular site, probably on the activity of DNA-dependent RNA polymerase. In addition, glucocorticoids may directly inhibit the synthesis of protein from ribosomal RNA in thymocytes and/or a metabolic step involving the utilization of precursors of RNA.

Morita and Munck have found that injection of cortisol into rats leads to decreased glucose uptake by thymus cells isolated two hours later. Cortisol added directly to cell suspensions of thymus tissue also decreased glucose uptake. From various studies Munck concludes that a primary physiologic action of glucocorticoids is to decrease glucose utilization by certain extrahepatic tissues. Suppression of glucose uptake may or may not be related to the decreased uptake or utilization of amino acids. There is also evidence to suggest that glucocorticoids may directly suppress transcription or synthesis of RNA from the DNA template. These effects have been observed by Kidson in seconds or minutes in suspensions of lymphoid cells. A decrease in mRNA synthesis would be expected to result in a decreased synthesis of protein as described in the chapter on genetic control of metabolism. Many of the mechanisms of action of steroid hormones have been explained by their action as a "repressor" or "de-repressor" of mRNA synthesis in their respective target tissues.

Glycolysis and Gluconeogenesis

ASHMORE, J., and MORGAN, D. Metabolic effects of adrenal glucocorticoid hormones. *In* Eisenstein, A.B., ed. *The Adrenal Cortex*. Boston, Little, Brown and Co., 1967, Chap. 7A, p. 249.

BALLARD, F.J., and HANSON, R.W. Phosphoenolpyruvate carboxykinase and pyruvate carboxylase in developing rat liver. *Biochem J*, 104:866, 1967.

HASLAM, J.M., and KREBS, H.A. The permeability of mitochondria to oxaloacetate and malate. *Biochem J*, 107:659, 1968.

JEFFERSON, L.S., EXTON, J.H., BUTCHER, R.W., SUTHERLAND, E.W., and PARK, C.R. Role of adenosine 3',5'-monophosphate in the effects of insulin and anti-insulin serum on liver metabolism. *J Biol Chem*, 243:1031, 1968.

KREBS, H.A. Renal gluconeogenesis. *In* Weber, G., ed. *Advances in Enzyme Regulation*. New York, Pergamon Press, 1963, Vol. 1, p. 385.

—— The regulation of the release of ketone bodies by the liver. *In* Weber, G., ed. *Advances in Enzyme Regulation*. New York, Pergamon Press, 1966, Vol. 4, p. 339.

LARDY, H.A. Gluconeogenesis: Pathways and hormonal regulation. *Harvey Lect*, 60:261, 1965.

—— PAETKAU, V., and WALTER, P. Paths of carbon in gluconeogenesis and lipogenesis: the role of mitochondria in supplying precursors of phosphoenolpyruvate. *Proc Nat Acad Sci USA*, 53:1410, 1965.

LEA, M.A., and WEBER, G. Role of enzymes in homeostasis. VIII. Inhibition of the activity of glycolytic enzymes by free fatty acids. *J Biol Chem*, 243:1096, 1968.

LONG, C.N.H., KATZIN, B., and FRY, E.G. The adrenal cortex and carbohydrate metabolism. *Endocrinology*, 26:309, 1940.

NEWSHOLME, E.A., and GEVERS, W. Control of glycolysis and gluconeogenesis in liver and kidney. *Vitamins Hormones*, 25:1. 1967.

RAY, P.D. Adrenal glucocorticoids and gluconeogenesis. *In* McKerns, K.W., ed. *Functions of the Adrenal Cortex*. New York, Appleton-Century-Crofts, 1968, Vol. 2, Chap. 28.

—— FOSTER, D.O., and LARDY, H.A. Mode of action of glucocorticoids. Stimulation of gluconeogenesis independent of synthesis de novo of enzymes. *J Biol Chem*, 239:3396, 1964.

SUTHERLAND, E.W., ØYE, I., and BUTCHER, R.W. The action of epinephrine and the role of the adenyl cyclase system in hormone action. *Recent Progr Hormone Res*, 21:623. 1965.

TAKEDA, Y., INOUE, H., HONJO, K., TANIOKA, H., and DAIKUHARA, Y.

Dietary response of various key enzymes related to glucose metabolism in normal and diabetic rat liver. *Biochim Biophys Acta*, 136:214, 1967.

WALTER, P., PAETKAU, V., and LARDY, H.A. Paths of carbon in gluconeogenesis and lipogenesis. 3. The role and regulation of mitochondrial processes involved in supplying precursors of phosphoenolpyruvate. *J Biol Chem*, 241:2523, 1966.

WEBER, G. Action of glucocorticoid hormone at the molecular level. *In* McKerns, K.W., ed. *Functions of the Adrenal Cortex*. New York, Appleton-Century-Crofts, 1968, Vol. 2, Chap. 27.

Adrenal Glucocorticoid Hormones and the Immune Response

GRANT, N. Metabolic effects of adrenal glucocorticoid hormones. *In* Eisenstein, A.B., ed. *The Adrenal Cortex*. Boston, Little, Brown and Co., 1967, Chap. 7B.

HAM, A. *Histology*. Philadelphia, J.B. Lippincott Co., 1965, pp. 257-350.

KIDSON, C. Cortisol in the regulation of RNA and protein synthesis. *Nature (London)*, 213:779, 1967.

MARKMAN, M.H., NAKAGAWA, S., and WHITE, A. Studies of the mode of action of adrenal steroids on lymphocytes. *Recent Progr Hormone Res*, 23:195, 1967.

MORITA, Y., and MUNCK, A. Effect of glucocorticoids *in vivo* and *in vitro* on net glucose uptake and amino acid incorporation by rat thymus cells. *Biochim Biophys Acta*, 93:150, 1964.

MUNCK, A. Metabolic site and time course of cortisol action on glucose uptake, lactic acid output, and glucose-6-phosphate levels of rat thymus cells *in vitro*. *J Biol Chem*, 243:1039, 1968.

WHITE, A., and GOLDSTEIN, A.L. Is the thymus an endocrine gland? Old problem, new data. *Perspect Biol Med*, 11:475, 1968.

4

Effects of Aldosterone on Electrolyte Homeostasis and Blood Pressure

FACTORS REGULATING ALDOSTERONE SECRETION

The enzyme renin, produced by the kidney, the vasoconstrictor peptide angiotensin II, and the steroid hormone aldosterone are important participants in electrolyte homeostasis and blood pressure control. Renin released from the kidneys acts on a plasma glycoprotein to form angiotensin I, which, in turn, is acted on by a converting enzyme to give the pressor peptide angiotensin II. Since angiotensin II is a potent vasoconstrictor substance, it can lead to an increase in blood pressure. In addition, angiotensin II stimulates the synthesis of aldosterone, probably from corticosterone, in the glomerular zone of the adrenal cortex. The renin-angiotensin system is operative at least in the dog, sheep, and human, but apparently not in the rat. Aldosterone stimulates the absorption of sodium in both the proximal and distal convoluted tubules of the kidney. This is usually accompanied by a parallel secretion of potassium and H^+. Aldosterone has a

57

one-hour latent period of action on the kidney. Rapid changes in sodium are generally attributed to effects on the glomerular filtration rate but the mechanism is unknown.

Regulation and Effect of Angiotensin II

Much evidence suggests that the renin-angiotensin system operates by a negative-feedback mechanism on the zona glomerulosa of the adrenal cortex to control the synthesis or release of aldosterone. That is to say, decreases in renal arterial pressure and/or renal blood flow, or possibly decreases in plasma sodium concentration, stimulate the release of renin. Renin, in turn, converts angiotensin I to angiotensin II.

The cytoplasm of the juxtaglomerular (JG) cells in the walls of the renal afferent arterioles contain granules rich in renin. The JG cells are in juxtaposition to the macula densa near the first segment of the distal convoluted tubule. These two cells actually interdigitate with one another, suggesting a functional relationship. These integrated cell units have been called the "juxtaglomerular apparatus." It seems likely that the macula densa is the sensor for the signal to renin release from the JG cells. The signal could conceivably be a decrease in the concentration of sodium or a decrease in arterial pressure and/or blood flow in the renal afferent arterioles, or both. There may be some separation of the vasoconstrictor effect of angiotensin II and its stimulatory effect on aldosterone secretion. Some experiments in the dog have shown that low levels of infusion of angiotensin II can stimulate secretion of aldosterone without a significant increase in blood pressure. Higher levels of infusion of angiotensin II increase blood pressure and stimulate release and synthesis of aldosterone, corticosterone, and cortisol. Under some circumstances, low levels of angiotensin increase blood pressure without an increase in aldosterone. The differences in response to angiotensin of the adrenal cortex as contrasted with the peripheral arterioles reflect the relative sensitivity of the target systems under varying physiologic conditions.

Other Factors in the Regulation of Aldosterone

Angiotensin II is one of the important mediators in the regulation of secretion of aldosterone from the zona glomerulosa of the adrenal cortex. However, ACTH may have a synergistic effect in the response and in addition can itself stimulate aldosterone synthesis. ACTH probably affects aldosterone synthesis by stimulating the formation of precursor steroids for aldosterone, such as progesterone and corticosterone.

Changes in the concentrations of Na^+ and K^+ of plasma also have a direct effect on the adrenal cortex to regulate aldosterone secretion. A decrease in the Na^+ level along with an increase in the K^+ level of the fluid perfusing the adrenal has been shown to increase aldosterone secretion. This can be an added stimulus to the response obtained when angiotensin II alone is perfused. Decreases in the Na^+ concentrations alone or increases in K^+ alone also stimulate aldosterone secretion, but appreciable changes in electrolyte concentrations are required to produce significant changes. However, selective increases in aldosterone secretion can be produced by sodium depletion without any change in plasma electrolyte levels. In regard to the influence of electrolyte changes on aldosterone synthesis, Sharma has demonstrated direct effects in vitro with adrenal glands from sheep, cattle, guinea pig, and human. The principal pathway of biosynthesis of aldosterone is apparently corticosterone to 18-hydroxycorticosterone and then to aldosterone (Chapter 2, Figure 3). Calçium increased the formation of 18-hydroxycorticosterone, whereas sodium greatly stimulated the conversion of 18-hydroxycorticosterone to 18-hydroxy-11-dehydrocorticosterone. This latter compound inhibits the step from corticosterone to 18-hydroxycorticosterone and thus could inhibit the main pathway of aldosterone synthesis. Also, Marusic and Mulrow found that adrenal mitochondria show enhanced corticosterone $\longrightarrow$ aldosterone when taken from animals on low Na^+ diets.

The central nervous system, via the hypothalamus, has an influence on the release of ACTH and thus has some effect on aldosterone secretion. Attempts to demonstrate an additional regulatory center in the diencephalon for the control of aldosterone secretion have not been entirely convincing.

Synthesis of Angiotensin II

The juxtaglomerular cells of the kidney contain large amounts of renin. When released from the kidney, this enzyme acts on a leucine-leucine bond of a glycoprotein contained in the alpha-2-globulin fraction of the plasma to release a decapeptide called angiotensin I. This glycoprotein substrate for renin is thought to originate in the liver. Angiotensin I is probably inactive. The plasma contains a large amount of a converting enzyme which cleaves histidine-leucine from the C terminal of the decapeptide to produce angiotensin II. These reactions are illustrated in Figure 1.

Renin is a labile enzyme, difficult to work with, and has not yet been obtained in a pure form. There are antigenic differences among renins in various animal species. In addition, hog renin, for example, will not attack human substrate. For these and other reasons the renin theory of hypertension has not been tested in humans. However, an antirenin has been produced in dogs. This antirenin neutralizes the activity of dog renin and will reduce the blood pressure to normal in dogs with renal hypertension, implicating the renin-angiotensin mechanism in this type of hypertension.

Normal human plasma and, in fact, most tissues of the body contain angiotensinase, which is able to degrade and inactivate angiotensins. There is no evidence that plasma angiotensinase has a physiologic role. However, the

Asp Arg Val Tyr Ileu His Pro Phe His Leu Leu Val Tyr Ser-Glycoprotein

Renin

Asp Arg Val Tyr Ileu His Pro Phe His Leu + Leu Val Tyr Ser-Glycoprotein

Converting enzyme
Cl^-

Asp Arg Val Tyr Ileu His Pro Phe + His Leu
(Angiotensin II)

Fig. 1. Formation of angiotensin II. The enzyme renin released from the kidney splits the leucine—leucine bond of a glycoprotein in the α-2-globulin fraction of the plasma to form a decapeptide called angiotensin I. A converting enzyme in the plasma cleaves histidine-leucine from the C terminal of angiotensin I to give angiotensin II.

cellular enzyme is no doubt important in the usual recovery from the angiotensin pressor response to the walls of the vascular system.

Negative Feedback in Aldosterone Secretion

This is illustrated in Figure 2. As mentioned previously, decreases in renal arteriolar pressure, renal blood flow, or sodium concentration may affect the juxtaglomerular apparatus in the renal afferent arterioles for the release of renin. The increased release of renin and an increase in the formation of angiotensin II by mechanisms described previously stimulate the release and synthesis of aldosterone. Presumably, any concomitant increased stimulus to secretion of corticosterone could soon be balanced by corticosterone inhibition of ACTH release. The increased aldosterone acts on the renal tubules causing increased reabsorption of sodium, usually with a parallel increase in K^+ or H^+ secretion. Water accompanies the sodium reabsorption. To account for chronic sodium and water retention some extraadrenal sodium-retaining factor must be present. This factor or functional response of the kidneys is unknown, but many patients with heart and circulatory disease or with liver disease have chronic sodium and water retention without demonstrable hypersecretion of aldosterone. In normal animals and man, retention of salt and water will increase circulating blood volume and perhaps cardiac output. In the presence of angiotensin, the hypervolemia (high blood volume) will tend to increase blood pressure and renal blood flow. A decreased rate of aldosterone metabolism arising because of a diseased liver, or a decrease in hepatic blood flow after hemorrhage or because blood flow is decreased in low-output heart failure may contribute to hyperaldosteronemia. These changes, then, could regulate renin release by the negative-feedback concept shown in Figure 2.

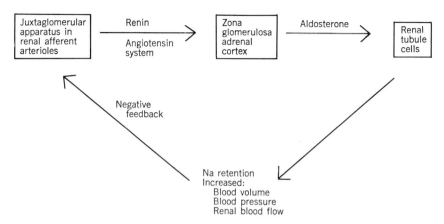

Fig. 2. Negative feedback in aldosterone secretion. These relationships are described in the text.

The renin-angiotensin system is a major mechanism for regulating aldosterone secretion. It appears to be necessary for the maintenance of functional activity of the adrenal zona glomerulosa along with ACTH. Angiotensin II may act primarily by a stimulation of pathways of steroidogenesis from corticosterone to aldosterone. The renin-angiotensin mechanism of homeostasis accounts at least in part for the hypersecretion of aldosterone following sodium depletion or in conditions affecting blood pressure or volume such as hemorrhage, heart failure, and pregnancy. In nephrotic syndromes, cirrhosis of the liver, and some hypertensive diseases, aldosterone is also increased. In addition, since angiotensin II has a powerful vasoconstrictor action on the smooth muscle of the vascular system, it probably plays an important role in hypertensive disease of renal origin.

MECHANISM OF ACTION OF ALDOSTERONE

The mineralocorticoid deoxycorticosterone is produced in larger amounts than aldosterone but has much less sodium-retaining activity. Aldosterone is the most active steroid hormone of the adrenal cortex involved in controlling the rate of reabsorption of sodium chloride from the proximal and distal convoluted tubules of the kidney. This effect is accompanied by enhanced secretion of potassium and hydrogen ions into the tubular urine. Water is passively absorbed with the salt. Aldosterone also has a role in regulating blood pressure, since low levels, as in Addison's disease, are associated with low blood pressure, and excess aldosterone, as in primary hyperaldosteronism due to adenoma of the glomerular zone of the adrenal, with high blood pressure. Aldosterone also stimulates sodium chloride absorption in the sweat and salivary glands and in the intestine. Thus, aldosterone is an essential hormone in the maintenance of normal electrolyte composition, circulatory volume, and blood pressure. With normal sodium intake, only about 100 to 150 micrograms per day are required for the average adult.

Some understanding of the mechanism of action of aldosterone on sodium transport has been achieved by the use of the isolated urinary bladder from the toad *Bufo marinus*. Regulation of sodium balance is a critical requirement of most multicellular organisms, and so aldosterone is produced by the adrenal cortex, as far as we know, by all vertebrates. Thus, not only does this hormone regulate the reabsorption of sodium chloride in the kidney of the human, it is essential to amphibians, including toads and frogs. The toad has a urinary bladder that conserves salt and water, thereby enabling this species to resist dehydration. It would seem that the mechanism of action of aldosterone on the epithelial cells of the toad urinary bladder is entirely comparable to the mechanism of action of aldosterone in the human kidney tubule. Thus, the toad urinary bladder has been used as a convenient and simpler experimental tool for studies of the effect of aldosterone and the mechanism by which aldosterone regulates salt retention. Some interesting concepts as to how aldosterone carries out its function have been developed by Edelman, Crabbé, and others.

According to Edelman, aldosterone specifically stimulates the transcription from nuclear DNA of a unique mRNA regulating the synthesis of a protein enzyme that is rate-limiting for the production of ATP by the mitochondria. Sodium is transported by an ATP-dependent process. These concepts are derived from the following observations. The administration of radioactive aldosterone to the toad leads to a concentration of the radioactive steroid in the nucleus of the epithelial cells of the urinary bladder of the toad. The administration of radioactive steroids such as estradiol, which have no effect on sodium retention in the epithelial cells, show uniform distribution of radioactivity throughout the epithelial cell. This suggests that the site of action of aldosterone is at the nucleus and correlates with the idea that certain hormones may stimulate transcription from a DNA molecule for the formation of a special messenger RNA (mRNA) concerned in the synthesis of an enzyme that is rate-limiting to metabolism.

Fitting in with this idea is the rather slow effect of aldosterone in inducing increased sodium retention. The effect of aldosterone on the toad bladder is not apparent until sixty to ninety minutes or so after its administration. In addition, it was found that inhibitors of protein synthesis, such as cycloheximide, inhibit the sodium-retaining effect of aldosterone. Cycloheximide inhibits protein synthesis by interfering with the transfer of amino acids from aminoacyl tRNA to the growing polypeptide chain. Thus, some rate-limiting protein enzyme seems to be involved in the mechanism of action of aldosterone. Puromycin, which seems to act by terminating the assembly of nascent polypeptide chains in the ribosomes, also inhibits the action of aldosterone. In addition, the administration of actinomycin D, which blocks transcription of DNA for the synthesis of mRNA by binding to the guanosine residues of DNA, also blocks the action of aldosterone. In this case, the inhibition is at the DNA-dependent site of mRNA synthesis.

The rate of total RNA synthesis was estimated by Edelman from the rate of incorporation of H^3-uridine into RNA in the toad bladder incubated in glass chambers in buffer solution. The rates of protein synthesis were estimated from the rate of incorporation of H^3-leucine or C^{14}-phenylalanine or C^{14}-serine into trichloroacetic acid or perchloric acid precipitates. The effects of the above-described protein or DNA inhibitors were studied in these isolated systems. The mechanism of action of aldosterone in accelerating the movement of sodium across the isolated toad bladder was correlated by a measurement of sodium estimated by an electrical conductivity method. The interruption of protein synthesis at three separate points in the biosynthetic pathway by the use of inhibitors prevented the action of aldosterone without inhibiting the baseline rate of sodium transport.

Such experiments, then, suggest that aldosterone stimulates or de-represses some nuclear DNA site for the synthesis of an mRNA, which in turn controls the synthesis of a protein enzyme essential to the mechanism of action of aldosterone. What this enzyme might be is not known. However, one clue is that if the bladder tissue is incubated with aldosterone in vitro in the absence of oxygen, there is no sodium-retaining effect of the steroid. This suggests that the unknown enzyme is one concerned in the metabolism of mitochondrial substrates concerned in the synthesis of ATP. It further suggests that there is an ATP-activated process for the aldosterone stimulus to sodium transport. These ideas are expressed graphically in Figure 3, which shows that on the urine side, sodium enters the epithelial cell, presumably by passive transport, and is pumped out of the epithelial cell into the interstitial fluid by an ATP-activated mechanism.

The hormone vasopressin, which is secreted from the posterior pituitary, also stimulates sodium retention. However, the mechanism seems to be different from that of aldosterone. Vasopressin stimulates active sodium transport across the isolated toad bladder by facilitating the entry of sodium into the epithelial cells by a mechanism not dependent upon ATP. Oxygen lack eliminates the response to aldosterone, but not the response to vasopressin. There is disagreement as to whether aldosterone acts to increase ATP concentrations or to affect the permeability of the target cells to sodium. Sharp and Leaf do not support the concept of an ATP-activated "pump" for the transport of sodium out of the epithelial cell. They argue that the aldosterone-induced protein may be a sodium-specific permease involved in bringing sodium into the cell from the urine side. Further studies are needed to resolve these differences.

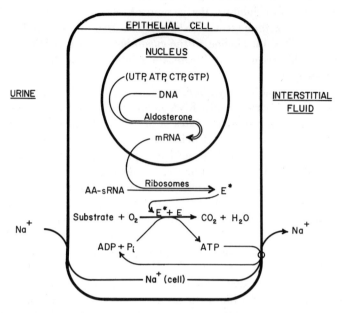

Fig. 3. The mechanism of action of aldosterone according to Edelman and associates. Aldosterone stimulates the transcription from nuclear DNA of an mRNA regulating the synthesis of a protein enzyme concerned in the production of ATP by the mitochondria. Na^+ is transported out of the cell by an ATP-dependent process. (From Edelman. *In* McKerns, ed. *Functions of the Adrenal Cortex*. Appleton-Century-Crofts, 1968, Vol. 1.)

PRIMARY AND SECONDARY HYPERALDOSTERONISM AND OTHER DISORDERS

Primary hyperaldosteronism is characterized by excess sodium retention with a corresponding potassium depletion. This condition is nearly always produced by an adenoma of the adrenal cortex, consisting of cells that resemble those of the glomerulosa and sometimes the fasciculata. The rest of the adrenal gland is usually of normal size and histology. The excess aldosterone is secreted by the adenoma. The disease is usually characterized by hypertension. There is excessive excretion of potassium in spite of low serum potassium. Most of the excessive loss of potassium and hydrogen ions is via the urine. The increased reabsorption of sodium with the passive absorption of water tends to increase the blood volume. The increase in blood volume is primarily due to an increase in plasma volume, and a low hematocrit is usual. Marked edema occurs when hemodynamic and fluid volume changes occur together. For reasons that are not yet clear, extracellular volume is not usually markedly increased in primary hyperaldosteronism. Primary hyperaldosteronism is characterized clinically by headaches, weakness, increased water intake, and increased urine volume, along with hypertension. The pulse rate is usually slow.

Certain abnormal conditions are characterized by a secondary stimulus to aldosterone secretion. Aldosterone secretion increases in hepatic cirrhosis with ascites, as plasma is lost from the vascular compartment. Here the activating stimulus may be through the renin-angiotensin-aldosterone mechanism described earlier, due to the decrease in plasma volume. An additional syndrome, that of congestive heart failure, may stimulate aldosterone secretion because of a disordered circulatory pattern. Again this may stimulate aldosterone through the renin-angiotensin system. A massive loss of protein as in nephrosis, along with leakage of plasma from the capillaries into tissue spaces, can produce a decrease in blood volume, which again can act as a stimulus to aldosterone secretion. In malignant forms of hypertension, aldosterone secretion is also increased. However, abnormalities due to aldosterone excess are not always seen. On the other hand, severe eyeground changes are seen. These are usually absent in primary hyperaldosteronism.

Factors Regulating Aldosterone Secretion

BLAIR-WEST, J.R., COGHLAN, J.P., DENTON, D.A., GODING, J.R., WINTOUR, M., and WRIGHT, R.D. The control of aldosterone secretion. *Recent Progr Hormone Res*, 19:311, 1963.

DAVIS, J.O. The regulation of aldosterone secretion. *In* Eisenstein, A.B., ed. *The Adrenal Cortex*. Boston, Little, Brown and Co., 1967, pp. 203-247.

——JOHNSTON, C.I., HOWARDS, S.S., and WRIGHT, F.S. Humoral factors in the regulation of renal sodium excretion. *Fed Proc*, 26:60, 1967.

GANONG, W.F., BIGLIERI, E.G., and MULROW, P.J. Mechanisms regulating adrenocortical secretion of aldosterone and glucocorticoids. *Recent Progr Hormone Res*, 22:381, 1966.

GROSS, F. Interrelationship of renal and adrenal hormones. *In* Martini, L., and Pecile, A., eds. *Hormonal Steroids*. New York, Academic Press, 1964, pp. 153-164.

——BRUNNER, H., and ZIEGLER, M. Renin-angiotensin system, aldosterone, and sodium balance. *Recent Progr Hormone Res*, 21:119,1965.

LEYSSAC, P.P. Intrarenal function of angiotensin. *Fed Proc*, 26:55, 1967.

MARUSIC, E.T., and MULROW, P.J. Stimulation of aldosterone biosynthesis in adrenal mitochondria by sodium depletion. *J Clin Invest*. 46:2101, 1967.

PEART, W.S. The functions for renin and angiotensin. *Recent Progr Hormone Res*, 21:73, 1965.

SHARMA, D. Discussion. *Recent Progr Hormone Res*, 22:425, 1966.

SKEGGS, L.T., LENTZ, K.E., GOULD, A.B., HOCHSTRASSER, H., and KAHN, J.R.R. Biochemistry and kinetics of the renin-angiotensin system. *Fed Proc*, 26:42, 1967.

TOBIAN, L. Renin release and its role in renal function and the control of salt balance and arterial pressure. *Fed Proc*, 26:48, 1967.

Mechanism of Action of Aldosterone

CRABBÉ, J. Site of action of aldosterone on the bladder of the toad. *Nature, (London)*, 200:787, 1963.

DE WEER, P., and CRABBÉ, J. The role of nucleic acids in the sodium-retaining action of aldosterone. *Biochim Biophys Acta*, 155:280, 1968.

EDELMAN, I. Aldosterone and sodium transport. *In* McKerns, K.W., ed. *Functions of the Adrenal Cortex*. New York, Appleton-Century-Crofts, 1968, Vol. 1, Chap. 4.

——BOGOROCH, R., and PORTER, G.A. Specific action of aldosterone on RNA synthesis. *Trans Ass Amer Physicians*, 77:307, 1964.

FALCHUK, M.Z., and SHARP, G.W.G. On the role of the tricarboxylic acid cycle in the stimulation of sodium transport by aldosterone. *Biochim Biophys Acta*, 153:706, 1968.

SHARP, G.W.G., and LEAF, A. Studies on the mode of action of aldosterone. *Recent Progr Hormone Res*, 22:431, 1966.

5

Hormone Regulation of Testes Function and Effects of Androgens

SPERMATOGENIC FUNCTION

The testes are composed of Leydig cells, which secrete the androgen steroids of the testes, and seminiferous tubules, which are concerned with the formation of the male gametes or spermatozoa. Spermatogenesis in the seminiferous tubules is a complicated series of events consisting of cell divisions and cell differentiations. The development and maturation of the spermatozoa proceed from the basal membrane of the tubule toward the lumen, where eventually spermatozoa are secreted into the duct. The differentiation of the primordial germ cells (gonocytes) proceeds to the primitive type A spermatogonia, possibly under the influence of testosterone or some other androgen. Several mitotic divisions are involved in the transformation through various forms of spermatocytes. Hormones do not seem to be required during these stages of mitotic division. The final spermatocytes undergo two maturation divisions to form spermatids. Testosterone may influence these steps. Final stages in the development of the spermatids are probably under the influence of follicle-stimulating hormone (FSH) from the anterior pituitary. This is the same hormone that stimulates the growth and function of follicles in the female. Thus, the completion of spermiogenesis (maturation of spermatids) requires FSH. The spermatogenic function of the testes and its regulation are extremely complicated. This subject has been elucidated by Steinberger and Steinberger.

BIOSYNTHESIS OF ANDROGENS IN THE TESTIS

The Leydig cells, which make up about 10 percent of the total testicular tissue, are the target cells that are stimulated by gonadotropins for an increased synthesis of androgens. The principal products secreted into the spermatic vein blood of the adult testis are testosterone and smaller amounts of 4-androstenedione and dehydroepiandrosterone. The major pathways for the synthesis of androgens are indicated in Figure 1. The formation of 5-pregnenolone from cholesterol occurs by reactions that have been previously described for the adrenal cortex and for the ovary.

A major pathway for the formation of androgens from 5-pregnenolone is apparently the Δ5 pathway from 5-pregnenolone to 17α-hydroxypregnenolone to dehydroepiandrosterone and thence to 4-androstenedione and testosterone. The reaction sequence from 5-pregnenolone to 4-androstenedione is the same as described for the reactions in the ovary and in the adrenal cortex. The other pathway illustrated in Figure 1 is 5-pregnenolone to progesterone and thence to 4-androstenedione. The pathways of androgen synthesis in the testis have been worked out. However, mitochondrial and microsomal function, metabolic pathways, the source of reducing equivalents, and mechanism of electron transport have not been studied as extensively as they have in the adrenal cortex. Presumably, similar mechanisms exist in the Leydig cells for the synthesis of androgens as occur for androgen synthesis in the adrenal cortex. Apparently, in the male at puberty there is an increase in activity and amount of the enzyme 17-dehydrogenase, which leads to a marked increase in formation of testosterone from 4-androstenedione. Testosterone is much more active as an androgenic steroid than is 4-androstenedione.

Concepts as to the regulation of the function of the testis are less developed than ideas about the regulation of the adrenal cortex and the ovary. The evidence suggests that similar mechanisms exist for the regulation of cell function and growth. Testicular steroid secretion can be stimulated by interstitial-cell-stimulating hormone (ICSH), known in female physiology as luteinizing hormone (LH), from the anterior pituitary and by the administration of other gonadotropins such as human chorionic gonadotropins (HCG). These hormones stimulate the formation and maintenance of the corpus luteum in the

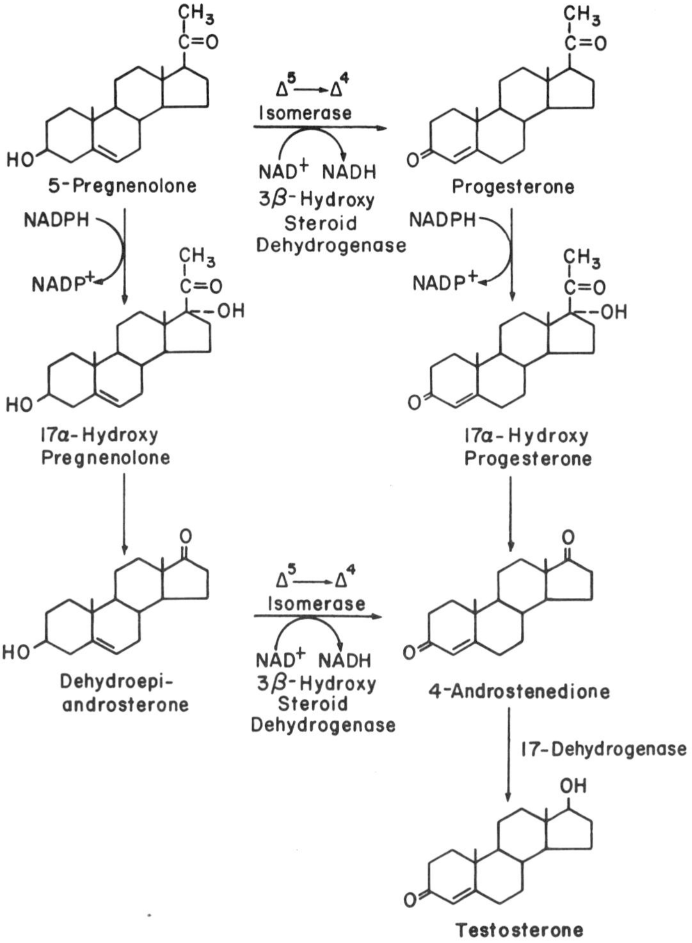

Fig. 1. Steroid synthesis in the testis. The major secretory products of the Leydig cells of the adult testis are testosterone, androstenedione, and dehydroepiandrosterone. The principal gonadotropic hormone that stimulates androgen synthesis is probably ICSH (LH).

female (luteotropic action). Possibly the principal gonadotropic hormone in the male regulating androgen secretion is ICSH. As in the case of the ovary and the adrenal cortex, the cyclic nucleotide 3′,5′-adenosine monophosphate (3′,5′-AMP) has been suggested as an intermediate in the mechanism of action of gonadotropin. This and other general concepts in the regulation of endocrine function are described in Chapter 11, on mechanisms of hormone action. Also, as suggested for the adrenal cortex and the ovary, the mitochondrial conversion of cholesterol to 5-pregnenolone has been suggested as a rate-limiting step, especially the 20-hydroxylation reaction of cholesterol. This step may be influenced by gonadotropins.

There may be species differences in the relative importance of pathways for biosynthesis of androgens. Connell and Eik-Nes have suggested that the $\Delta 5$ pathway indicated in Figure 1 is the principal pathway in the canine testis, whereas Dorfman and associates suggest that the pathway of progesterone to 17α-hydroxyprogesterone to testosterone is more important in man and other primates.

ANDROGEN-INDUCED GROWTH
AND EFFECTS OF ANABOLIC STEROIDS

It has been appreciated for a long time that there is some association of the male gonad and androgenic compounds with the muscle mass of the body and the development of sex characteristics. Eunuchs who have had their testes removed before puberty have reduced muscle growth and strength, whereas precocious puberty due to hyperactivity of the testis may be accompanied by marked development of skeletal muscle relative to age. In addition, castration of the human male before puberty leads to other characteristic differences from the normal. Height is increased, with the lower limbs disproportionately long owing to retarded ossification of the epiphyses of the long bones. The voice does not deepen, nor is the larynx prominent. Face and body hair fail to grow, though hair may be abundant on the head. Sex drive is low and the penis is infantile. The administration of androgenic steroids to the castrate male will overcome many of these deficiencies.

The development of secondary sex characteristics in the male at puberty is due to an increase in androgen secretion from the interstitial cells of the testis. These androgens are largely testosterone, androsterone, and dehydroepiandrosterone. Testosterone is about six times more androgenic than androsterone and even more active than dehydroepiandrosterone. There is also an increased ratio of testosterone to the other androgens at puberty. Androgens are also secreted by the reticular zone of the adrenal cortex; and virilization, especially noticeable in the female, can occur with increased secretion of androgens from the adrenal cortex. This is known as the "adrenogenital syndrome" and can occur because of a genetic deficiency of the 21-hydroxylase enzyme, or because of a relative lack of other enzymes concerned in the formation of 17α-hydroxycorticosterone. Substrate steroid is thus diverted to the formation of androgens.

The androgens, then, are anabolic, increasing tissue growth and muscle mass, with an increased retention of nitrogen, potassium, phosphorus, and calcium. However, androgens are not the only anabolic steroids. Growth hormone, estrogens, thyroid hormone, and insulin, as well as other trophic hormones such as adrenocorticotropin and gonadotropin, increase growth in their target organs. This growth effect is generally more limited to certain tissues than in the case of androgens. Estrogens, for example, stimulate the growth of the uterus and the female genital tract and, along with other hormones, increase the development of the breast. Estrogens are antagonistic to the action of the androgens; and to some extent, development of the secondary sex characteristics is regulated by the balance between these two classes of hormones. For example, androgen-induced growth of the prostate is suppressed by estrogen, and estrogens are thus commonly administered for carcinoma of the prostate.

The effect of androgen in inducing an increase in the size of androgen-sensitive tissues is not always due to an increase in the number of cells or quantity of DNA. For example, androgen-induced enlargement of the levator ani muscles and kidneys of castrated mice, or the masseter muscles of castrated guinea pigs, is due to hypertrophy rather than to cell division. The androgen-induced increase in the size of all skeletal muscle is believed to be caused by hypertrophy rather than an increase in the number of muscle fibers. The hypertrophy of the comb after androgen treatment of the capon is caused by an increased synthesis of hyaluronic acid and water retention.

Much work has been carried out in an attempt to obtain steroid compounds that have an anabolic effect on skeletal muscle with a minimum androgenic effect or stimulus to secondary sex characteristics. Evaluations have often been carried out on castrated young male rats by comparing the increase in the ratio of the weight of the levator ani muscle to the weight of the ventral prostate or seminal vesicle. The increase in the weight of the levator ani is taken to be the anabolic response and the increase in weight of the ventral prostate or seminal vesicle as the androgenic effect. Many steroids have been synthesized that are more anabolic than androgenic as compared with testosterone. There is some question as to the validity of this technique as a means of distinguishing anabolic from androgenic effects in the first place. Furthermore, differences in experimental procedure and in the potency ratings of compounds used add to the problem of characterizing anabolic compounds by this particular procedure. Anabolic compounds should have a nitrogen-sparing effect. Nitrogen balance and other studies have also been carried out with animals and in clinical studies to test various compounds.

In spite of the limitations and difficulties of the methods, many so-called anabolic steroids have been synthesized and made available for clinical use. They have been used in cases of underweight for which no endocrine or other detectable cause has been determined. In these cases, anabolic steroids have been given along with an optimal protein diet. Protein deficiency resulting from chronic infections, such as pulmonary tuberculosis, has also been treated with anabolic steroids. Synthetic anabolic compounds have been used in the treatment of osteoporosis, muscular dystrophy, diabetic retinopathy, and cirrhosis of the liver. A list of many anabolic compounds available, their clinical use, and side effects has been compiled by Kruskemper.

In spite of the widespread use of anabolic steroids there is little understanding of their mechanism of action. In fact, the mechanism of action of the natural androgens is not understood, though much evidence indicates that increases in ribonucleic acid and protein are part of the androgen-induced growth and differentiation of sexual organs of the male.

The growth and development of the male accessory glands are dependent on androgens, and the rat prostate has been a convenient organ to study these effects. Growth of this gland involves hypertrophy of the epithelial cells, formation of secretory products, and hyperplasia of various cellular elements with an increase in the total amount of DNA. Castration of the adult rat leads to a rapid decline of these parameters in the ventral prostate. Treatment with physiologic amounts of androgens restores DNA and RNA content, along with growth of the ventral prostate. Williams-Ashman and co-workers have found that daily treatment of castrated rats with large amounts of androgens results in a massive but transitory increase in DNA polymerase activity. There was increased incorporation of nucleotide precursors into DNA in in vitro systems. Increases in nuclear RNA polymerase were found to precede the increased activity of DNA polymerase. These experiments suggest, but do not prove, that androgens have some effect on stimulating or unmasking genetic DNA synthesis of RNA. An increase in mRNA would increase protein synthesis. An increase in protein enzyme synthesis would increase the metabolic activity of the cell and, in turn, could lead to an increase in cell replication and DNA synthesis. Hormonal regulation of metabolic activity and cell replication are discussed further in Chapter 10.

There is an indication that at least part of the growth effect of androgens in some males with delayed sexual development may be due to increased release of growth hormone. Martin and associates have suggested that the growth-promoting effects of androgens in dwarfed children may be mediated through stimulation of the pituitary gland.

Ciba Foundation Colloquium on Endocrinology. *Endocrinology of the Testis.* Boston, Little, Brown and Co., 1967, Vol. 16.

COFFEY, D.S., SHIMAZAKI, J., and WILLIAMS-ASHMAN, H.G. Polymerization of deoxyribonucleotides in relation to androgen-induced prostatic growth. *Arch Biochem*, 124:184, 1968.

CONNELL, G.M., and EIK-NES, K.B. Metabolism leading to the formation of testosterone in the rabbit and dog testis. *In* McKerns, K.W., ed. *The Gonads.* Part 3: Functions of the Testes, New York, Appleton-Century-Crofts, 1969, Chap. 17.

DORFMAN, R.I., FORCHIELLI, E., and GUT, M. Androgen biosynthesis and related studies. *Recent Progr Hormone Res*, 19:251, 1963.

KRUSKEMPER, H.L. *Anabolic Steroids.* New York, Academic Press, 1968.

LIPSETT, M.B., WILSON, H., KIRSCHNER, M.A., KORENMAN, S.G., FISHMAN, L.M., SARFATY, G.A., and BARDIN, C.W. Studies on Leydig cell physiology and pathology: secretion and metabolism of testosterone. *Recent Progr Hormone Res*, 22:245, 1966.

MARTIN, L.G., CLARK, J.W., and CONNOR, T.B. Growth hormone secretion enhanced by androgens. *J Clin Endocr*, 28:425, 1968.

McKERNS, K.W., ed. *The Gonads*. Part 3: Functions of the Testes. New York, Appleton-Century-Crofts, 1969.

STEINBERGER, E., and STEINBERGER, A. The spermatogenic function of the testes. *In* McKerns, K.W., ed. *The Gonads*. Part 3: Functions of the Testes. New York, Appleton-Century-Crofts, 1969, Chap. 22.

WILLIAMS-ASHMAN, H.G., LIAO, S., HANCOCK, R.L., JURKOWITZ, J., and SILVERMAN, D.A. Testicular hormones and the synthesis of ribonucleic acids and proteins in the prostate gland. *Recent Progr Hormone Res*, 20:247, 1964.

6

Regulation of Ovarian Processes

CYCLIC CHANGES
IN GROWTH AND STEROIDOGENESIS

After menstruation, the next cycle is concerned with the growth of the graafian follicles and, in the human, the complete maturation of usually only one, with the release of an ovum and the formation of a corpus luteum. The cellular growth changes and the changing pattern of steroidogenesis are under the influence of gonadotropins released from the pars distalis of the hypophysis (anterior pituitary).

At the beginning of the cycle, the levels of estrogens and progesterones are low. The cycle begins with the release of follicle-stimulating hormone (FSH) from the anterior pituitary, which stimulates cellular replication and steroidogenesis. In the early part of the menstrual cycle, under the influence of FSH the granulosa cell layers of the primordial follicles proliferate and differentiate to produce the graafian follicles. In terms of steroid function in the early part of

75

the menstrual cycle, the synthesis and secretion of estrogen are due primarily to FSH stimulus of the theca interna cells, which proliferate and enlarge under the influence of FSH. The growth of the follicle, then, is due to proliferation of granulosa cells and cells of the theca interna and distention of the cavity of the follicle with fluid. The estrogens secreted by the theca cells stimulate cell replication of the endometrium of the uterus and increase the electrical and contractile activity of the myometrium of the uterus. Estrogens also stimulate the vagina, breast, and adipose tissue.

Just prior to the midpoint of the menstrual cycle, there is a marked increase in the amount of luteinizing hormone (LH) released from the anterior pituitary. LH, in conjunction with FSH, stimulates additional cell replication and steroidogenesis, the release of the ovum, and the formation of a corpus luteum. The formation of the corpus luteum which proceeds after ovulation contributes most of the progesterone of the second half of the menstrual cycle. Luteotropic hormone (LTH or prolactin) has a role in the maintenance of the corpus luteum. In the absence of pregnancy, the average life of the corpus luteum is about fourteen days. In the rabbit and rat, and possibly in the human and other species, LH stimulates an increase in 20α-steroid dehydrogenase (or 20β-steroid dehydrogenase) in the interstitial tissue, which lowers the activity of progesterone by reducing the 20-keto group. This is apparently one factor signifying a decrease in function of the corpus luteum in the absence of implantation of a fertilized ovum.

In the first half of the menstrual cycle, estrogen is the growth hormone of the endometrium in that it stimulates cellular proliferation. Under the influence of progesterone in the second half of the menstrual cycle, the endometrium of the uterus becomes secretory. The cells of the endometrial glands hypertrophy, and there is a marked increase in the blood supply in the stroma due to an increase in arterioles. The endometrium becomes receptive to the implantation of a fertilized ovum. R. M. Wynn's *Cellular Biology of the Uterus* is a comprehensive treatment of the structure and regulation of the uterus.

STEROID SYNTHESIS IN THE OVARY

The principal cells of the ovary involved in steroid synthesis are the theca and granulosa of the follicle and those of the corpus luteum derived from these cells. These cells are able to synthesize cholesterol from acetate and store it as fatty acid esters of the 3-hydroxyl group of cholesterol. The conversion of cholesterol to 5-pregnenolone is a reaction common to all endocrine tissues that secrete steroid hormones. These reactions are the same as those described for the adrenal cortex. They consist of a 20α-hydroxylation of the side chain of cholesterol followed by a 22ξ-hydroxylation by two specific hydroxylase enzymes. This is followed by a cleavage of the side chain of cholesterol by a desmolase enzyme yielding 5-pregnenolone and isocaproic acid, which derives from the isocaproaldehyde of the side chain. Again, as in the case of the adrenal cortex, the hydroxylation reactions require molecular oxygen and reducing equivalents from NADPH. The gonadotropic hormones not only regulate the availability of reducing equivalents for hydroxylation and reductive reactions in the ovary but also regulate cell replication of various cells in the ovary.

Metabolic pathways for the production of reducing equivalents such as NADPH, the coupling of NADPH to mitochondrial and microsomal electron transport for steroid hydroxylations, or reductive reactions have not been fully studied in the ovary. However, processes similar to those described for the adrenal cortex probably exist in the ovary. For example, there is some evidence that glucose-6-phosphate dehydrogenase and the pentose phosphate pathway provide reducing equivalents for steroid hydroxylations and reducing processes in the ovary. Ribose sugars derived from this pathway may also be rate-limiting to the synthesis of RNA. Gonadotropins may control the rate of metabolism of glucose-6-phosphate by stimulating the activity of glucose-6-phosphate dehydrogenase. These and other hypotheses as to the regulation of function in the ovary have been reviewed by McKerns.

It must be kept in mind that the first half of the menstrual cycle, or the follicular phase, is concerned primarily with the secretion of estrogens. The rise in progesterones occurs in the second, or luteal, phase due mostly to the formation of a corpus luteum. These patterns of steroidogenesis agree with the concept that estrogens are largely secretory products of cells of the theca interna, and progesterone is secreted largely from the granulosa cells of the late follicle phase, about midcycle, and from cells of the corpus luteum derived from granulosa cells.

The principal reactions that occur in the transformation of 5-pregnenolone to progesterone and other progestational compounds and, via androgens, to estrogens are given in Figure 1. The reactions of the theca interna are shown on the left side of the figure. In the theca cells estrogen production is for the most part through pregnenolone. The granulosa cells and the corpus luteum have an active series of enzymes for the conversion of 5-pregnenolone to progesterone, and thus progesterone is a major secretory product. To a lesser extent, 17α-hydroxyprogesterone is secreted. There is a more limited conversion of progestins to estrogens by these cells.

The formation of progesterone from 5-pregnenolone involves the removal of hydrogen from the 3-hydroxyl group of 5-pregnenolone by 3β-hydroxysteroid dehydrogenase, which utilizes NAD^+ as the hydrogen acceptor. NADH can be reoxidized by the mitochondria and also possibly by extramitochondrial lactic dehydrogenase where pyruvate is reduced to lactate. The oxidation of the 3-hydroxyl by 3β-hydroxysteroid dehydrogenase is followed by a shift in the double bond from the 5 position to the 4 position catalyzed by an enzyme or an enzyme complex called Δ5-Δ4 isomerase. Both 5-pregnenolone and progesterone

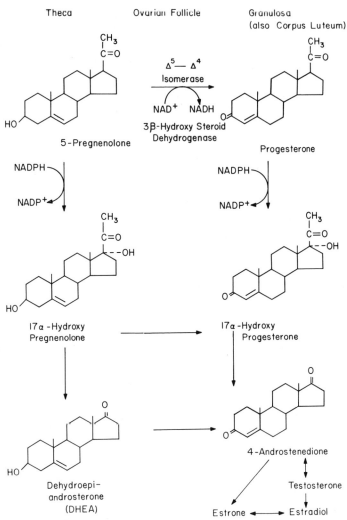

Fig. 1. Pathways for the synthesis of progesterones, androgens, and estrogens by cells of the ovary. In the first half of the menstrual cycle (follicular phase) estrogens are synthesized mainly by the pathway 5-pregnenolone to 17α-hydroxypregnenolone to dehydro-epiandrosterone. This latter androgen is converted by a specific dehydrogenase and by an isomerase to 4-androstenedione. Estrone is formed by aromatization of 4-androstenedione. Other reactions of estrogen synthesis from androgens are shown in Figure 2. Granulosa cells of the follicle, just prior to ovulation, and the corpus luteum, after ovulation, secrete progesterones largely since they have enzymes able to convert 5-pregnenolone to progesterone. Some estrogen is also produced by these cells.

can be hydroxylated in the 17α position, forming the corresponding 17α-hydroxy steroid. A desmolase enzyme is able to cleave the 17β side chain of pregnenolone or progesterone to give either dehydroepiandrosterone or 4-androstenedione respectively. Androstenedione is converted to estrone by a process known as aromatization. Before dehydroepiandrosterone is aromatized to estrogen it is converted to its 3-keto derivative (5-androstene-3,17-dione) by the enzyme $\Delta 5$, 3β-hydroxysteroid dehydrogenase (3β-hydroxysteroid dehydrogenase). However, a separate $\Delta 5,3$-ketosteroid isomerase probably exists for the conversion of 5-androstene-3,17-dione to 4-androstenedione.

The aromatization of androgens to estrogens occurs largely in the microsomes of the cell and, again, requires NADPH and molecular oxygen. These reactions are shown in Figure 2. A 17-dehydrogenase enzyme can lead to an interconversion of androstenedione and testosterone and the interconversion of estrone and estradiol.

MAINTENANCE OF THE CORPUS LUTEUM

The corpus luteum is essential for the maintenance of pregnancy, at least during the first trimester of human gestation. An essential factor in the functional persistence of the corpus luteum in human pregnancy is the

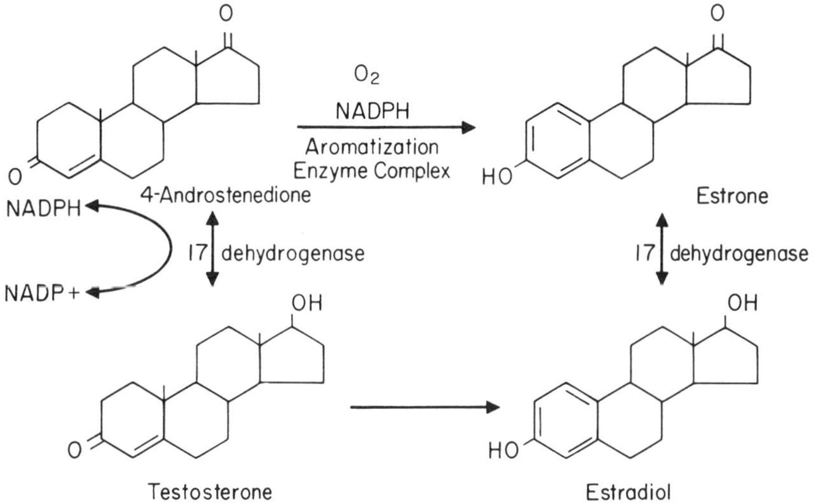

Fig. 2. Aromatization of androgens to estrogens. Androstenedione derived from dehydro-epiandrosterone or from 17α-hydroxyprogesterone is converted to the corresponding estrogen by the formation of an aromatic ring structure in ring A of the steroid. In this process, the 19-methyl is removed, the 3-keto group is reduced, and two hydrogens are removed from ring A. A 17-dehydrogenase enzyme can reduce the 17-keto or oxidize the 17-hydroxyl group of androgens or estrogens.

production and secretion of chorionic gonadotropin by the chorion cells of the placenta.

The corpus luteum of early human pregnancy provides estrogens for the growth of the uterus and progesterones. Progesterones are believed to have a relaxing effect upon the uterus, which suppresses contractions. After the first trimester, the production of estrogens and progesterones is taken over by the placenta itself.

In most mammals other than primates, the ovary provides the estrogens and progesterones. This involves both persistent corpora lutea or the constant formation of new corpora lutea, and presumably also functional follicular activity. Several recent studies in animals have suggested theories as to the maintenance of the corpus luteum. It is not known to what extent these might apply to the human. In essence, it is a question of whether factors operate to maintain the corpus luteum which would otherwise degenerate, or whether the corpus luteum would survive indefinitely were there not factors operating to cause its breakdown. In certain species, in the absence of implantation, a luteolytic factor from the uterus has been postulated to cause the lysis of the corpora lutea. On the other hand, it has been suggested that implanatation leads to various hormonal mechanisms which are involved in maintaining the corpora lutea.

Lysis of the Corpus Luteum by a Uterine Luteolytic Factor

It has been postulated that in certain animal species a specific internal secretion from the mucosa of the uterus is responsible for shortening the life of the corpus luteum in the absence of implantation of a fertilized ovum or ova. At least it is known that removal of the uterus (hysterectomy) can extend the life-span of functional corpora lutea in guinea pigs, rats, rabbits, cows, sheep, and pigs. This extension is approximately equal to the length of the normal gestation period of the species. On the other hand, hysterectomy has little or no effect on the duration of the corpora lutea in the ferret and the rhesus monkey. In the human, the menstrual cycle is slightly prolonged if hysterectomy is carried out three to four days after the ovulation period. This may imply that there is some effect of the uterus in the human on corpus luteum function. If so, its significance is not known.

In the first series of animals named above, where the uterine lytic stimulus is stronger than the luteotropic stimulus, the action of the early embryo implantation is thought to be antiluteolytic rather than luteotropic. In other words, the implantation is considered to suppress the factors involved in lysis of the corpus luteum, rather than providing additional gonadotropin for its stimulation. When the uterus is under progesterone stimulus it is thought that it produces a luteolytic substance which causes luteal regression in the absence of an embryo. Estrogen seems to depress the luteolytic stimulus. The humoral substance that seems to be involved in lysis of the corpus luteum in certain species has not been isolated.

Some evidence for the existence of such a uterine luteolytic factor has been obtained by Shomberg. Granulosa cells from sow ovaries at the preestrus stage were maintained in tissue culture. Flushing of the uterine horns of sows was carried out with tissue culture medium. It was found that during days 12 through 18 of the estrus cycle the uterus of the sow produced a high molecular weight substance that caused a morphologic luteolytic effect on the granulosa cells.

Hypophyseal and Other Factors in Luteolysis

Malven has reviewed the current knowledge on the process of luteolysis in the laboratory rat. In this review, luteolysis is considered to be a two-stage process—functional and structural. Functional luteolysis involves a decrease in the secretion of progesterone into the blood, coinciding with an increase in the enzyme 20α-steroid dehydrogenase. This enzyme causes a substantial decrease in the activity of progesterone by converting the 20-keto group to the 20α-hydroxyl. Structural luteolysis has been defined as morphologic regression of the corpus luteum. In the laboratory rat, hypophysectomy leads to functional luteolysis but retards structural luteolysis.

The intravenous injection of luteinizing hormone (LH) can acutely stimulate progesterone secretion. Prolactin (luteotropic hormone or LTH) does not seem to stimulate progesterone synthesis. On the other hand, prolactin, but not LH, maintains functional corpora lutea after hypophysectomy. A possible explanation for the effect of prolactin in maintaining the corpus luteum has been suggested by Wiest and Kidwell. Prolactin can inhibit the activity or synthesiss of 20α-hydroxysteroid dehydrogenase and thus prevent the catabolism of progesterone to the less active 20α-hydroxy derivative of progesterone. According to the suggestions of Malven, termination of functional corpora lutea may involve three possibilities: marked decrease in prolactin secretion, an effect of uterine or hypophyseal factors in antagonizing the luteotropic action of prolactin, or absence of a placental luteotropin. They may all operate simultaneously to cause functional luteolysis.

Wiest and Kidwell have also studied factors involved in the maintenance of the corpus luteum. They have been concerned with the function of the dehydrogenase enzymes 3β-hydroxysteroid dehydrogenase and glucose-6-phosphate dehydrogenase, which act to increase progesterone synthesis, and of 20α-hydroxydehydrogenase, which acts to decrease progesterone in the laboratory rat. The administration of FSH and LH stimulates steroidogenesis at least in part by increasing the amounts of glucose-6-phosphate dehydrogenase and 3β-hydroxysteroid dehydrogenase. These enzymes also increase in activity during the functional period in the estrus cycle and in pregnancy. The finding that these enzymes increase is supporting evidence that they do have an important role in ovarian function. After ovulation and in the absence of pregnancy, the enzyme 20α-hydroxysteroid dehydrogenase increases concomitantly with increases in plasma levels of 20α-hydroxy derivative of progesterone.

At the beginning of the estrus cycle in the rat, FSH stimulates follicle development with an increase in estrogen and an increase in glucose-6-phosphate dehydrogenase and the pentose phosphate pathway. At this time, the low plasma levels of progesterone permit the release of pituitary LH necessary to initiate ovulation. LH further stimulates the pentose phosphate pathway and increases other enzymes concerned in the synthesis of progesterone, such as 3β-hydroxy-steroid dehydrogenase. In an unmated rat, after ovulation the corpus luteum regresses rapidly owing to a lack of luteotropic hormone (LTH), as well as to an effect of LH in increasing 20α-hydroxysteroid dehydrogenase. However, when cervical stimulation occurs, either artificially or by mating, LTH released from the pituitary maintains the new corpus luteum both functionally and morphologically for several days. An increase in 20α-hydroxysteroid dehydrogenase activity is prevented through the action of LTH and a lack of sufficient LH, so that progesterone reduction to the 20α-hydroxy compound is retarded. If nidation occurs, luteotropins from the placenta relieve the pituitary of this function. The activity of 20α-hydroxysteroid dehydrogenase continues to be suppressed, allowing continued secretion of progesterone. Luteotropic hormone secretion from the placenta declines prior to parturition. This leads to a drop in the synthesis of progesterone with a subsequent partial removal of the inhibition to LH release. The declining level of LTH and the increasing level of LH initiate 20α-hydroxysteroid dehydrogenase activity. Thus, a shift of progesterone to the relatively inactive 20α-hydroxy compound occurs, and delivery of the fetuses follows shortly.

Such mechanisms of control of the function of the corpus luteum may have relevance to the human and other primates in the maintenance of the corpus luteum of early pregnancy. However, after about the first trimester (about ninety days), ovarian steroid function in the human is replaced by de novo production of progesterone by the placenta, and by the aromatization of androgens reaching the placenta from the maternal and fetal adrenal cortex, where they are converted to estrogens.

Hilliard, Spies, and Sawyer have reviewed the hormonal factors regulating estrus, ovulation, pregnancy, and pseudopregnancy in the rabbit. The rabbit is a reflex ovulator. That is to say, coitus in the rabbit in estrus leads to a stimulus to the hypothalamus which initiates a release of LH from the anterior pituitary. The initial release of LH stimulates the interstitial tissue of the ovary with an increased production of the 20α-hydroxy derivative of progesterone. This preovulatory release of 20α-hydroxy derivative of progesterone prevents progesterone inhibition of LH, which continues to be released and insures ovulation. The ovary at this period becomes relatively insensitive to LH, apparently owing to a depletion of cholesterol stores for steroid synthesis. At this time, prolactin (LTH) is released from the anterior pituitary causing hypertrophy of the interstitial cells, which then accumulate cholesterol and regain their sensitivity to LH. Prolactin thus maintains the morphology of the interstitial tissue and its capacity to secrete steroids. Apparently, in this species at least, estrogen secretion from the ovarian follicles is essential to maintain luteal development and function. The level of estrogen is regulated by the uterus. The uterus during gestation metabolizes less estrogen, and this sparing effect makes more available to sustain the corpora lutea. If implantation does not occur, the rate of metabolism by the nonpregnant uterus is such that insufficient estrogen is available to stimulate progesterone synthesis from the corpora lutea. When the level of progesterone falls, LH from the anterior pituitary is released, the 20α-hydroxy derivative of progesterone increases, and luteolysis occurs.

BLAND, K.P., and DONOVAN, B.T. The uterus and the control of ovarian function. *In* McLaren, A., ed. *Advances in Reproductive Physiology.* New York, Academic Press, 1966, Vol. 1, pp. 179-214.

EIK-NES, K.B. The effects of gonadotrophins on the secretion of steroids by the testis and the ovary. *Physiol Rev,* 44:609, 1964.

GINTHER, O.J. Local utero-ovarian relationships. *J Anim Sci,* 26:578, 1967.

HILLIARD, J., SPIES, H.G., and SAWYER, C.H. Hormonal factors regulating ovarian cholesterol mobilization and progestin secretion in intact and hypophysectomized rabbits. *In* McKerns, K.W., ed. *The Gonads.* Part I: Functions of the Ovaries. New York, Appleton-Century-Crofts, 1969, Chap. 3.

MAHESH, V.B., and GREENBLATT, R.B. Steroid secretions of the normal and polycystic ovary. *Recent Progr Hormone Res,* 20:341, 1964.

MALVEN, P.V. Hypophyseal regulation of luteolysis in the rat. *In* McKerns, K.W., ed. *The Gonads.* Part 1: Functions of the Ovaries. New York, Appleton-Century-Crofts, 1969, Chap. 14.

McKERNS, K.W. Genetic, biochemical, and hormonal mechanisms in the regulation of uterine metabolism. *In* Wynn, R.M., ed. *Cellular Biology of the Uterus.* New York, Appleton-Century-Crofts, 1967, Chap. 5.

—— Studies on the regulation of ovarian function. *In* McKerns, K.W., ed. *The Gonads.* Part 1: Functions of the Ovaries. New York, Appleton-Century-Crofts, 1969, Chap. 6.

ROTHSCHILD, I. The corpus luteum—hypophysis relationship. The luteolytic effect of luteinizing hormone (LH) in the rat. *Acta Endocr (Kobenhavn),* 49:107, 1965.

RYAN, K.J., and AINSWORTH, L. Comparative aspects of steroid hormones in reproduction. *In* Benirschke, K., ed. *Comparative Aspects of Reproductive Failure*. New York, Springer-Verlag, 1967.

——and SMITH, O.W. Biogenesis of steroid hormones in the human ovary. *Recent Progr Hormone Res*, 21:367, 1965.

SAVARD, K., MARSH, J.M., and RICE, B.F. Gonadotropins and ovarian steroidogenesis. *Recent Progr Hormone Res*, 21:285, 1965.

SHOMBERG, D.W. The concept of a uterine luteolytic hormone. *In* McKerns, K.W., ed. *The Gonads*. Part 1: Functions of the Ovaries. New York, Appleton-Century-Crofts, 1969, Chap. 15.

SHORT, R.V. Ovarian steroid synthesis and secretion *in vivo*. *Recent Progr Hormone Res*, 20:203, 1964.

——Reproduction. *Ann Rev Physiol*, 29:373:1967.

WIEST, W.G., and KIDWELL, W.R. The regulation of progesterone secretion by ovarian dehydrogenases. *In* McKerns, K.W., ed. *The Gonads*. Part 1: Functions of the Ovaries. New York, Appleton-Century-Crofts, 1969, Chap. 11.

WYNN, R.M., ed. *Cellular Biology of the Uterus*. New York, Appleton-Century-Crofts, 1967.

7

Hormone Function in the Human Placenta and Fetal Adrenal Cortex

HORMONE SYNTHESIS BY THE HUMAN PLACENTA

Soon after implantation of the trophoblast, the growth of the chorion cells leads to secretion of the protein hormone chorionic gonadotropin. This hormone stimulates the ovary and, along with pituitary hormones and other factors, maintains estrogen and progesterone secretion and aids in the maintenance of the corpus luteum of pregnancy. By about the end of the first trimester (ninety days), pregnancy can be maintained independent of ovarian function. That is to say, the placenta provides the necessary estrogens and progesterones for the maintenance of pregnancy. Chorionic gonadotropin reaches a peak value of from 40,000 to 100,000 IU per 24 hours by the fiftieth to seventieth day of gestation. Secretion of the hormone decreases during the next few weeks to around 4,000 to 11,000 IU for the remainder of pregnancy. This time of decreasing synthesis of chorionic gonadotropin represents a period of full functional capacity for the synthesis of progesterones and estrogens by the placenta and a decreasing importance of the corpus luteum for steroid synthesis in human pregnancy.

Animal species other than primates are dependent on ovarian function throughout pregnancy in regard to the production of estrogen and progesterone. When the human placenta becomes fully functional in the synthesis of steroid hormones, the steroids secreted are principally progesterone, 5-pregnenolone, large amounts of estriol, smaller amounts of 20α- and 20β-hydroxy derivative of progesterone, estrone, and estradiol. The progestational steroids are synthesized de novo (that is, from acetate or cholesterol) by the placenta, but estrogens are derived by aromatization of androgen precursors from the fetal or maternal adrenals.

Many other hormones, both polypeptide and steroid, have been isolated from the placenta, but the placenta contains large amounts of maternal and fetal blood and may, in addition, concentrate certain steroids, so that it becomes difficult to say whether they are actually synthesized in the placenta. It seems likely that a placental lactogenic hormone which also has many of the properties of growth hormone is produced by the placenta. The function of this polypeptide hormone is not understood.

Little can be said about the regulation of the growth and function of the placenta. Neither the pituitary nor the ovary has been demonstrated to exert any direct control over placental function. There is a possible reciprocal relationship between chorionic gonadotropin and estrogen-progesterone levels in the placenta, but this has not been proven.

The de novo synthesis of progesterone from cholesterol by the placenta is essential to the maintenance of human pregnancy after the first trimester when ovarian function declines. The placenta has enzymes for the synthesis of cholesterol from acetate and for the production of 5-pregnenolone from cholesterol. As far as is known, these transformations are similar to, or the same as, the enzymatic mechanisms found in other endocrine tissues. Presumably, the formation of 5-pregnenolone occurs largely in the mitochondria. As previously described for the ovary, the formation of 5-pregnenolone involves hydroxylations at the 20 and 22 positions of the cholesterol side chain, followed by a cleavage of the side chain between the 20 and 22 positions by a desmolase enzyme. The formation of progesterone from 5-pregnenolone involves the removal of the hydrogen from the 3-hydroxyl by 3β-hydroxysteroid dehydrogenase utilizing NAD^+ as the hydrogen acceptor and a shift of the double bond from the 5 to the 4 position by the Δ5,Δ4-isomerase enzyme.

The placenta is also very active in converting androgenic steroids, such as androstenedione, dehydroepiandrosterone, and 16α-hydroxydehydroepiandrosterone, to phenolic estrogens. This general series of reactions is termed "aromatization of C-19 steroids." The enzymes concerned in these reactions are found largely in the microsomal fraction of the syncytiotrophoblast of the placenta. They require NADPH and oxygen. The aromatization reactions and the possible sources of reducing equivalents (NADPH) are probably the same as those described for the ovary. Unlike the ovary, the placenta does not synthesize estrogens from acetate via cholesterol through pregnenolone or progesterone, but is dependent on androgens derived from the fetal adrenal cortex or from the maternal adrenal for conversion to estrogens. The fetal adrenal cortex secretes largely $\Delta5$-androgens such as dehydroepiandrosterone and 16α-hydroxydehydroepiandrosterone. The latter compound is converted to estriol by the human placenta. Since the placenta does not have a 16α-hydroxylase, the secretion of estriol reflects the formation of the 16α-hydroxylated androgen precursor from the fetal adrenal cortex. Part of the secretion of $\Delta5$-androgens by the fetal adrenal cortex represents the conversion of 5-pregnenolone reaching the fetus from placental secretion. This is in addition to the de novo synthesis of $\Delta5$-androgens by the fetal adrenal cortex.

THE FETAL ADRENAL CORTEX

The fetal adrenal cortex is intriguing because of a marked hypertrophy of a "fetal zone" between the medulla and the reticular zone of the definitive cortex. During early fetal development the adrenal glands grow more rapidly than the rest of the body, reaching a maximum size about the fourth month of human pregnancy. The fetal zone regresses rapidly after birth.

The mechanism of the development of the fetal zone is unclear. The fetal zone is small or absent in anencephalic fetuses. This may be due to a lack of hypothalamic corticotropin-releasing factor or minimal development of the adenohypophysis in the anencephalic infant. Thus, the development of the fetal adrenal zone requires a functional adenohypophysis under hypothalamic control. It is possible that 3β-hydroxysteroid dehydrogenase in the fetal adrenal cortex is inhibited in early fetal life by estrogen, 5-pregnenolone, or progesterone from the corpus luteum, leading to a shift in the pattern of steroid synthesis, hypertrophy of the reticularlike fetal zone, and an increase in androgen secretion.

In the first half of gestation the human fetal adrenal has a deficiency of 3β-hydroxysteroid dehydrogenase and $\Delta5,\Delta4$-isomerase. The deficiency or inhibition of these enzymes results in the secretion of $\Delta5$-androgens such as dehydroepiandrosterone. The large amount of androgens produced by the fetal adrenal cortex represents a function of the fetal zone to form androgens from 5-pregnenolone. The fetal adrenal is capable of de novo synthesis of 5-pregnenolone as well as being able to convert 5-pregnenolone from the placenta. Pregnenolone is hydroxylated at the 17 position to form 17α-hydroxypregnenolone, and the side chain is cleaved by a desmolase enzyme to yield dehydroepiandrosterone (DHEA) by reactions described for the theca cells of the ovary. DHEA may be further hydroxylated to give the 16α-hydroxy derivative.

Even by midpregnancy the fetal adrenal still utilizes progesterone from the placenta for the most part for the synthesis of glucocorticoids such as corticosterone, and mineralocorticoids such as deoxycorticosterone and aldosterone. The ready availability of progesterone from the placenta may bypass the necessity for de novo synthesis of glucocorticoids. Glucocorticoids and mineralocorticoids are available to the fetus from the maternal adrenal cortex. That the fetus receives glucorticoids and mineralocorticoids from the maternal adrenal has been shown by transfer studies using radioactive steroids and by the fact that anencephalic infants can come to term without a functional adrenal cortex.

In later pregnancy, fetal adrenal cortex undoubtedly shows an increased ability to form progesterone from 5-pregnenolone and an ability for the de novo synthesis of glucocorticoids and aldosterone. It is deduced that this ability is developed in the fetal adrenal cortex from the fact that the neonate must have a self-sufficient mechanism for the production of glucocorticoids and mineralocorticoids in order to survive.

INTERRELATIONS OF STEROID HORMONE METABOLISM IN THE FETUS AND PLACENTA

Although the placenta is not capable of synthesizing estrogens de novo from acetate or cholesterol, it does have a great capacity to carry out aromatization of C-19 androgenic steroids to estrogens. These enzymes are located in the microsomes of the placenta. The androgen precursors for estrogen biosynthesis in the placenta come from both the maternal and the fetal adrenal cortex. As mentioned previously, the human fetal adrenal cortex secretes large quantities of Δ5-androgens such as dehydroepiandrosterone and its 16α-hydroxy derivative. These steroids are secreted largely as the sulfate ester of the 3-hydroxy. Since the placenta does not have a 16α-hydroxylation mechanism, the major precursor for estriol synthesis in the placenta is the 16α-hydroxylated androgen, 16α-hydroxy-dehydoepiandosterone. The placenta contains a very active sulfatase enzyme system. The placental hydrolysis of circulating androgen sulfates is followed by rapid aromatization as indicated in Figure 1. Thus, estriol is derived for the most part from an androgen precursor from the fetal adrenal. The concentration of estriol in the urine during pregnancy parallels the size of the fetus and the capacity of the fetal adrenals to secrete 16α-hydroxydehydroepiandrosterone. This relationship explains the greatly diminishing estriol secretions in women pregnant with anencephalic fetuses which have an atrophic

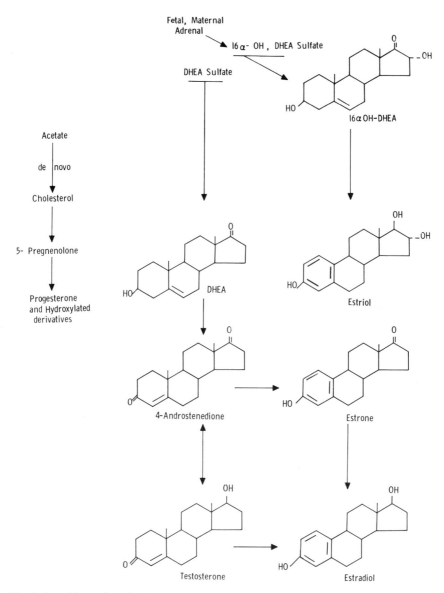

Fig. 1. Steroid reactions in the human placenta after the first trimester. These reactions bypass the dependency for estrogens and progesterones from the ovary. Progesterone and hydroxylated derivatives can be synthesized de novo. Androgens from the fetal or maternal adrenal cortex provide precursors for the synthesis of estrogens. Dehydroepiandrosterone (DHEA) is converted to androstenedione and to estrone and estradiol. Estriol synthesis is mostly a reflection of the capacity of the fetal adrenal cortex to provide the precursor as 16α-hydroxy DHEA.

fetal adrenal cortex. In this condition, apparently androstenedione and dehydroepiandrosterone are supplied by the maternal adrenal cortex in quantities sufficient to provide these precursors for aromatization to estrone and estradiol in amounts adequate to maintain pregnancy.

Large quantities of progesterone are secreted by the placenta into both fetal and maternal organisms where the steroid is extensively metabolized. The synthesis of progesterone in the placenta can take place de novo from acetate, as indicated in Figure 1. Progesterone secreted by the placenta can be converted by the fetal adrenal into 6β-, 16α-, 17α-, and 20α-hydroxyprogesterones. The placenta can reconvert 20α-hydroxyprogesterone back to progesterone, thus conserving progesterone.

The fetal adrenal is capable of synthesizing glucocorticoids using the progesterone from the placenta as precursor. These glucocorticoids include

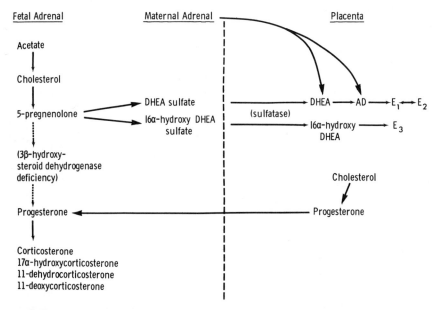

Fig. 2. Relationships of steroid synthesis in the fetal adrenal cortex and the placenta in humans. The adrenal cortex of the fetus can synthesize 5-pregnenolone. However, even by midpregnancy there is little conversion to progesterone. Pregnenolone is diverted to androgens such as dehydroepiandrosterone (DHEA) and 16α-hydroxy DHEA. These androgens are aromatized to estrogens by the placenta: DHEA to androstenedione (AD) to estrone (E_1) and estradiol (E_2); 16α-hydroxy DHEA to estriol (E_3). The adrenal cortex of the mother can also provide DHEA and AD. Androgens are transported in the blood as sulfate esters. The placenta has sulfatases to remove the esters.

After the first trimester, the placenta can synthesize progesterone and various hydroxylated derivatives from cholesterol in increasing quantities as gestation proceeds, to maintain pregnancy. Some of the progesterone that passes through the placenta to the fetal circulation can be used for the synthesis of glucocorticoids by the fetal adrenal cortex. However, during fetal life, adequate glucocorticoid and mineralocorticoid can be provided by the adrenal cortex of the mother.

corticosterone, deoxycorticosterone, 11-dehydrocorticosterone, and 17α-hy-droxycorticosterone. These are secreted both as the free compounds and as the sulfate esters. Steroid relationships between the fetal adrenal and the placenta are summarized in Figure 2.

BLOCH, E. Fetal adrenal cortex: Function and steroidogenesis. *In* McKerns, K.W., ed. *Functions of the Adrenal Cortex*. New York, Appleton-Century-Crofts, 1968, Vol. 2, Chap. 19.

Ciba Foundation Study Group No. 27. *The Human Adrenal Cortex: Its Function Throughout Life*. Boston, Little, Brown and Co., 1967.

JOHANNISSON, E. The foetal adrenal cortex in the human. *Acta Endocr (Kobenhavn)* 58: Suppl. 130:7, 1968.

RYAN, K.J., and AINSWORTH, L. Comparative aspects of steroid hormones in reproduction. *In* Benirschke, K., ed. *Comparative Aspects of Reproductive Failure*, New York, Springer-Verlag, 1967.

SOLOMON, S., BIRD, C.E., LING, W., IWAMIYA, M., and YOUNG, P.C.M. Formation and metabolism of steroids in the fetus and placenta. *Recent Progr Hormone Res*, 23:297, 1967.

8

Catabolism and Inactivation of Steroid Hormones by the Liver and Kidney

All of the steroid-producing glands secrete into the bloodstream, which carries the steroids to the liver and kidney where they are eventually inactivated by a series of reactions. The metabolites are excreted in the urine, largely conjugated as sulfate esters or β-glucosiduronates. The role of the liver in this inactivation is emphasized by the fact that the rate of disappearance of cortisol from the blood is greatly decreased in liver disease. A normal half-life of cortisol ($11\beta,17\alpha21$-trihydroxy-4-pregnene-3,20-dione), for example, is about 100 minutes. There is a great host of metabolites excreted in the urine; however, there are only certain major reactions of the hormones other than conjugation possible. These include (1) the reduction of the Δ^4 3-keto function, (2) reduction of the 20-keto group, (3) cleavage of the side chain to give 17-keto steroids, and (4) oxidation of the 17β-hydroxyl group in C_{19} steroids. These reactions for three classes of steroids are shown in Figure 1 and will be discussed in detail.

The liver can reduce the Δ^4 3-keto function of corticoids, androgens, and progesterone. The irreversible reduction of the double bond (introduction of H to C-4 and C-5) is generally followed by the reduction of the 3-keto group (to the 3-hydroxyl). These two reactions can be considered together and called *ring A reduction*. The loss of the Δ^4 3-keto grouping largely inactivates the biologic

93

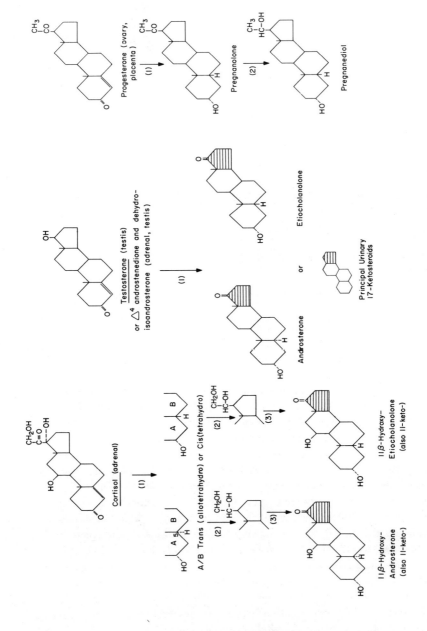

Fig. 1. Major reactions in the metabolism of glucocorticoids, androgens, and progesterones by liver enzymes.

potency of the corticoids and progesterones and greatly reduces the activity of the androgens. In the reduction of the 4,5 unsaturation, the hydrogen at C-5 can be introduced in either the α or β orientation. The enzyme concerned with the β reducation at C-5 of cortisone or cortisol is predominant in man. The enzyme of the liver that carry out these C-5 reductions require NADPH and are concentrated in the microsomes (5α enzyme) or cytoplasm (5β enzyme) of the liver cells. Reduction of the 3-keto in man is usually to a 3α-hydroxysteroid with either NADPH or NADH as cofactor.

There is very little interconversion of the 11-oxygen function of the 5β-H derivative of cortisol and cortisone (tetrahydrocortisol and tetrahydrocortisone); whereas in the 5α-H series, the 11-keto group is readily reduced to give the 11β-hydroxy derivative (allotetrahydrocortisol) as the major product. These tetrahydro derivatives are found in the urine largely as the glucosiduronates with trace amounts as sulfates. Thus, four urinary excretion products of cortisol are possible as a result of the formation of either A/B *trans* (5α-H, allotetrahydro) or A/B *cis* (5β-H, tetrahydro) compounds with a keto or hydroxyl group at carbon 11. The compounds with an intact dihydroxyacetone side chain appear to be the major urinary excretion products of cortisol (20 to 40 percent). These compounds are given in Figure 2.

In man, cortisol is quantitatively the major secretory product of the adrenal cortex. However, there is a reversible oxidation-reduction reaction between cortisol and cortisone occurring mainly in the liver with NADP$^+$ as the more effective cofactor. Cortisone has about two-thirds the glucocorticoid activity of cortisol and a half-life of only 30 minutes. In addition, cortisone, unlike cortisol, has little or no suppressive effect on ACTH secretion. Thus, this reversible system is the principal determinant of the level of circulating cortisol. The 11β oxidation-reduction enzyme system is influenced by the level of thyroid hormones in the blood. Hyperthyroidism stimulates the oxidative reaction to cortisone. In addition, much of the cortisol is bound to a gamma globulin fraction of the blood plasma. This cortisol-binding protein increases under the influence of estrogen, and in pregnancy approximately 85 percent of the cortisol is protein-bound. The rate of liver inactivation of protein-bound cortisol is less than for free cortisol. Cortisol is apparently only active as the free steroid in its function as a glucocorticoid and in its ability to suppress ACTH synthesis and release.

Progesterone is secreted by the ovary for the most part during the luteal phase and by the placenta during pregnancy. It also undergoes reduction of the Δ^4 3-keto function to afford mainly the *cis* (5β-H) pregnane compounds (e.g., pregnanolone in Fig. 1).

The androgens, derived mainly from the adrenal and the testis, are again reduced in similar fashion, with the Δ^4 3-keto group yielding either the A/B *trans* compound (androsterone) or the A/B *cis* compound (etiocholanolone). The 17β-hydroxyl group of testosterone can be oxidized to the 17-ketone. Androgens are excreted as glucosiduronates or sulfates.

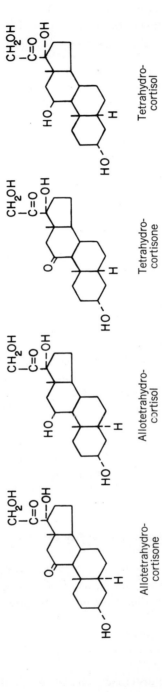

Fig. 2. Cortisol metabolism by reduction of the Δ^4 3-keto positions to give A/B *trans* (allotetrahydro) or A/B *cis* (tetrahydro) compounds.

96

The quantitatively minor compounds that are secreted by the adrenal cortex in the human—aldosterone, 11-deoxycorticosterone, and corticosterone— for the most part are reduced to the corresponding A/B *cis* (tetrahydro) compounds, as shown in Figure 3, but both *cis* or *trans* compounds are possible.

Aldosterone is biologically inactivated by the liver, largely by reduction of the 20-ketone and by reduction of the Δ^4 3 keto function to form the tetrahydro derivative. This compound is excreted by the kidney as the glucosiduronate of the C-3 hydroxyl group.

Further catabolic changes can occur in compounds that have a C-17 side chain by reduction of the 20-keto group. This is illustrated at (2) in Figure 1. In this transformation the kidney as well as the liver plays a role. The enzymes responsible for this are 20-keto reductases which are concentrated in kidney and liver microsomes and require NADPH as the coenzyme. The 20-keto group of tetrahydrocortisone and tetrahydrocortisol may be reduced, giving either 20β-hydroxy or 20α-hydroxy derivatives. There is a 20-keto reductase for cortisol different from the one for progesterone derivatives. The reduction of the 20-keto group of cortisol can also occur before Δ^4 3-keto reduction. In fact, the

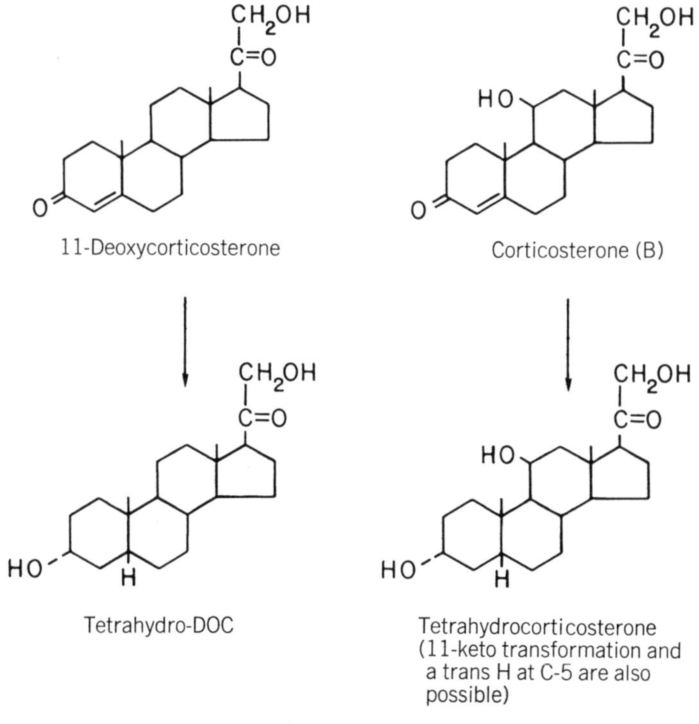

CH$_2$OH
C=O

11-Deoxycorticosterone

CH$_2$OH
C=O

Corticosterone (B)

CH$_2$OH
C=O

Tetrahydro-DOC

CH$_2$OH
C=O

Tetrahydrocorticosterone
(11-keto transformation and
a trans H at C-5 are also
possible)

Fig. 3. Metabolism of deoxycorticosterone and corticosterone by the liver to A/B *cis* (tetrahydro) compounds by reduction of the Δ^4 3-keto positions.

CH₂OH ... (figure)

| Cortolone | β-Cortolone | Cortol | β-Cortol |

Fig. 4. Reduction of the 20-keto group of tetrahydrocortisone to give 20α-hydroxy (cortolone) or 20β-hydroxy (β-cortolone) compounds. The corresponding reduction of tetrahydrocortisol to 20α- or 20β compounds is also shown. The reduction of the 20-keto group of compounds such as cortisol can also occur before Δ^4 3-keto reduction.

principal route for the production of cortolone is via the formation of a 20α-hydroxy derivative of cortisol, which is then reduced at the Δ^4 3-keto positions. These compounds are shown in Figure 4.

These highly hydroxylated steroids appear to be the next major urinary end products of the catabolism of cortisol and cortisone in humans after the tetrahydro derivatives. Some 20 to 30 percent of an intravenous dose of cortisol can be recovered in the urine as these four derivatives.

The 20-keto-group of ring-A-reduced (*cis*) metabolites of progesterone and 17α-hydroxyprogesterone can also be reduced to give pregnanediols and pregnanetriols. (It has been found that following the intravenous injection of 4-C^{14}-progesterone to human subjects with bile fistula, approximately 30 percent of the injected radioactivity was recovered in the bile and 50 percent in the urine.) The pregnanes excreted in human urine and in bile include the major metabolic excretory products of progesterone—pregnanediol, pregnanolone (not reduced in the 20-keto position), and, to a lesser extent, allopregnanediol (*trans*). These compounds are illustrated in Figure 5.

The adrenal secretes only small quantities of progesterone and 17α-hydroxyprogesterone into the bloodstream. Men, or women in the follicular phase of the menstrual cycle or after menopause, have a urinary excretion of pregnanediol of only approximately 1 mg per day. The principal endocrine tissue that secretes progesterone in the normal female is the ovary during the luteal

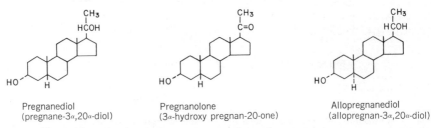

| Pregnanediol | Pregnanolone | Allopregnanediol |
| (pregnane-3α,20α-diol) | (3α-hydroxy pregnan-20-one) | (allopregnan-3α,20α-diol) |

Fig. 5. The major metabolic excretory products of progesterone.

phase. The placenta produces very large quantities of progesterone, especially during late pregnancy, and thus large amounts of progesterone metabolites are found in the urine during late pregnancy.

Small amounts of pregnanetriols derived from 17-α-hydroxyprogesterone may be found in the urine and in the bile (especially in late pregnancy), such as 5β-pregnane-3α,17α,20α-triol, shown in Figure 6.

Additional secretory products in the pregnane series may include trace amounts of 11-keto and 11-hydroxy derivatives of these compounds, especially in congenital adrenal hyperplasia.

Further metabolic transformations of the steroid hormones by liver enzymes include oxidative cleavage of the side chain of corticoids and, to a limited extent, of the pregnanetriols to give 17-ketosteroids. The 17-ketosteroids arising from cortisol catabolism are 11-keto- and 11β-hydroxyandrosterone, and 11-keto- and 11β-hydroxyetiocholanolone. Each accounts for about 3 percent of the urinary products recovered from an administered dose of radioactive cortisol. As was mentioned earlier, the two principal 17-ketosteroids arising from the catabolism of the androgens (e.g., testosterone, Δ^4-androstenedione, and dehydroepiandrosterone) are androsterone and etiocholanolone. The latter compounds are excreted largely as glucosiduronates. In some patients large amounts of dehydroepiandrosterone can be produced by the adrenal and excreted unchanged without ring A reduction, conjugated principally as the sulfate. The principal source of three 17-ketosteroids, dehydroepiandrosterone, etiocholanolone, and androsterone is the adrenal gland. The quantitative separation and measurement of these 11-deoxyandrogen derivatives is often an important diagnostic guide to the detection of virilizing adrenal tumors.

Estrogens are excreted in the urine largely as sulfate esters or as glucosiduronates of estrone, estradiol, estriol, and 2-hydroxyestrone. Estradiol is the principal estrogen secreted by the follicles of the ovary. Estradiol is rapidly oxidized in the liver, and possibly in other tissues, to estrone and more slowly reduced back to estradiol. Estrone may be hydroxylated at the C-16 and C-2 positions. Hydroxylation at C-16 leads to the formation of estriol. Hydroxylation at C-2 forms 2-hydroxyesterone, which can be further metabolized by

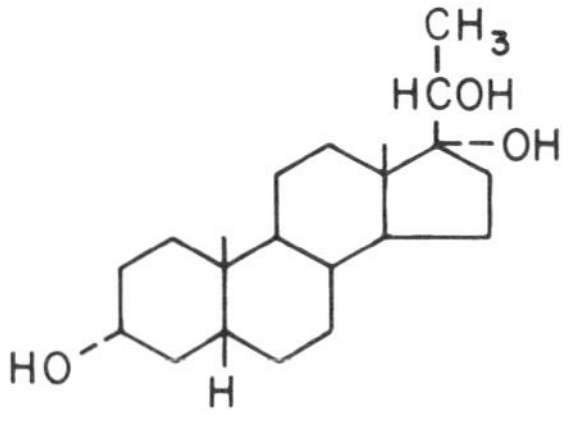

5β-Pregnane-3α,17α,20α-triol

Fig. 6. Pregnanetriol is found in the urine and bile, especially in late pregnancy. This compound is derived from 17α-hydroxyprogesterone via 17α-hydroxypregnanolone.

methylation of the C-2 phenolic group. These relationships are shown in Figure 7. These compounds are the major estrogen metabolites found in the urine, with estrone and 2-hydroxyestrone the principal metabolites in normal subjects.

About half of the estrogen secreted appears in the bile, and part of these products undergo enterohepatic circulation. Little is known of the possible products excreted by the gastrointestinal tract. Most analytic methods account for only about 40 percent of estrogen injected in metabolic studies. In most clinical studies, only estrone, estradiol, and estriol are measured in the urine, although 2-hydroxyestrone is one of the most important metabolites. It has been ignored because of the difficulty in its measurement. Lisboa and Diczfalusy have reported and characterized a total of 24 estrogen excretion products in the urine.

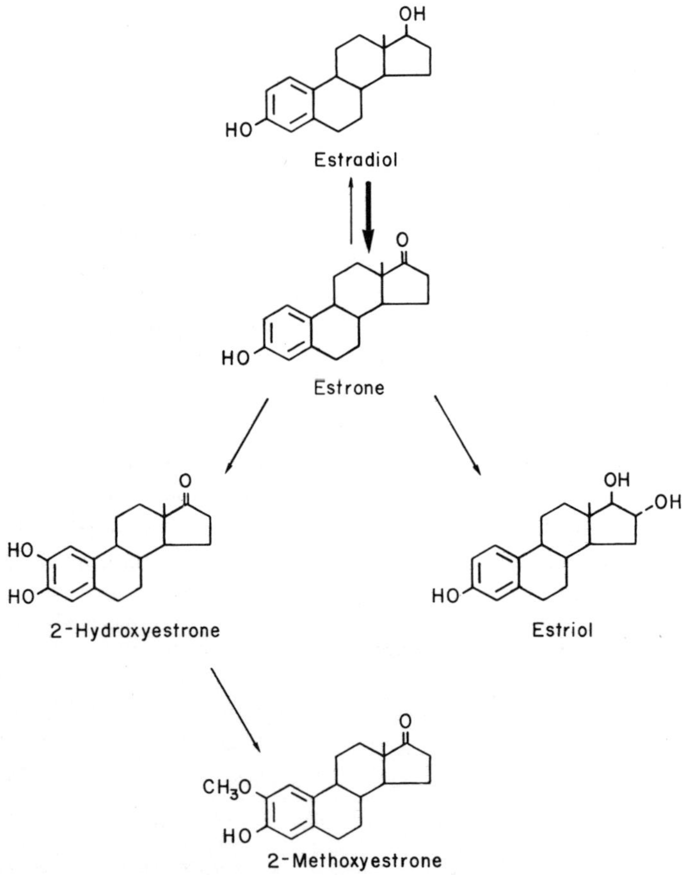

Fig. 7. Some metabolic products of estradiol formed in the liver in the nonpregnant female.

MEASUREMENT OF STEROID METABOLITES
AND ESTIMATE OF ADRENAL FUNCTION

An estimate of function of endocrines that secrete steroid hormones can be made by measuring the concentration of certain steroid metabolites in blood plasma or urine. Along with clinical observations, these measurements are useful guides to diagnosis and therapy. A few examples will be given for the estimation of function of the adrenal cortex.

A general decreased or increased function of the adrenal cortex can be assessed by the amounts of 17-hydroxycorticosteroids (17-OHCS) excreted in the urine. These metabolites of cortisol are the tetrahydro derivatives shown in Figure 2 and represent 20 to 30 percent of the cortisol that is secreted. These compounds are often measured by a phenylhydrazine—sulphuric acid reaction developed by Porter and Silber, after solvent extraction of urine that has been subjected to enzyme hydrolysis. The tetrahydro derivatives of cortisol can also be measured in blood plasma by the Porter-Silber reaction or modifications of it.

Changes in cortisol secretion may be primary at the adrenal level, or secondary due to changes in secretion of ACTH from the anterior pituitary. For example, adrenocortical insufficiency (Addison's disease) may be due to acute or chronic failure or atrophy as a result of trauma, infection, or hemorrhage; or it may be secondary to ACTH deficiency. Similarly, a chronic excess secretion of cortisol, as in Cushing's syndrome, may be due to a basophilic adenoma of the pituitary or to another source of ACTH, such as from an ectopic tumor. On the other hand, Cushing's syndrome may be the result of excess cortisol secretion from adrenocortical neoplasm.

To aid in the diagnosis, the measurement of 17-OCHS can be made by comparing the basal level of excretion with levels found after stimulation or suppression of the adrenal cortex. The response of the adrenal cortex to administered ACTH is made after several complete 24-hour urine collections are obtained and the amount of 17-hydroxycorticosteroid determined. Usually ACTH (25-50 USP units) is then given as a constant, intravenous infusion over 8 hours. A 24-hour collection of urine is assayed. ACTH may be repeated on the second day. Primary failure of the adrenal cortex is indicated by a failure to increase the secretion of 17-OHCS. In secondary adrenal insufficiency the excretion is only slightly increased, but it increases further by the second day. In pituitary-dependent hypercortisolism, patients show a three- to five-fold increase in excretion of 17-OHCS over their already high levels. Most cases of Cushing's syndrome due to adrenocortical carcinoma fail to respond to ACTH.

Glucocorticoids suppress the secretion of ACTH from the anterior pituitary. Certain synthetic glucocorticoids such as Δ^1-9α-fluorohydrocortisone or its 16α-methyl derivative, dexamethasone, are such potent suppressors that they contribute little to the assay of 17-OHCS, and are thus used in ACTH suppression tests. For example, patients with a pituitary-dependent hypercortisolism can be suppressed with 2 to 8 mg of dexamethasone every six hours. Cushing's syndrome due to adrenocortical tumors or the ACTH from non-pituitary tumors (ectopic) is resistant to suppression.

Another agent used to test pituitary-adrenal responsiveness is Metopirone (2-methyl-1,2-bis-[3-pyridyl]-1-propanone), SU-4885 (Ciba). This compound is a specific inhibitor of 11β-hydroxylase activity. Cortisol synthesis is inhibited, and thus the secretion of ACTH from the anterior pituitary is increased in normal subjects. The immediate precursor of cortisol (substance S, lacking the 11-hydroxyl group) is increased and can be measured as an 17-OHCS. Cushing's syndrome due to an andrenocortical neoplasm fails to respond to Metopirone. If the Cushing's disease is controlled by pituitary ACTH, the patient responds with an increase in 17-OHCS. In patients having an ectopic source of ACTH, response to Metopirone will occur only where the adrenal cortex is not already maximally stimulated by ACTH.

Increases in androgen secretion can occur from the adrenal cortex owing to virilizing adrenal tumors or to congenital adrenal hyperplasia. The latter hyperplasia may be due to a deficiency of 21-hydroxylase or other enzymes concerned in the synthesis of cortisol. The deficiency in cortisol increases the secretion of ACTH, leading to enlargement of the adrenal cortex. Because of the enzyme deficiencies, steroid substrate is diverted to the synthesis of androgens. Virilism is, of course, especially noticeable in the female and may be characterized by hirsutism, menstrual disorders, clitoral hypertrophy, masculine body appearance, and deepening of the voice. The 17-ketosteroids of the urine are elevated and if these are fractionated, dehydroepiandrosterone, androsterone, and etiocholanolone are seen to be increased. The measurement of 17-ketosteroids in plasma or urine may be carried out in conjunction with similar stimulating or suppressing tests described previously to assess whether a tumor is involved, or if there is an enzyme deficiency in the adrenal. Surgical removal of virilizing adrenal tumors can be carried out with good prognosis if they are well encapsulated and show minimal signs of malignancy. Adrenal hyperplasia, due to a deficiency of 21-hydroxylase or other enzymes of steroid synthesis, can be treated by giving cortisol or some other glucocorticoid. Glucocorticoids suppress the secretion of ACTH from the anterior pituitary, reduce the hyperplasia of the adrenal cortex, and aid in restoring the normal spectrum of steroids.

BAULIEU, E.E., PEILLON, F., and MIGEON, C.J. Adrenogenital syndrome. *In* Eisenstein, A.B., ed. *The Adrenal Cortex*. Boston, Little, Brown and Co., 1967, Chap. 15.
BROWN, J.B., and MATTHEW, G.D. The application of urinary estrogen

measurements to problems in gynecology. *Recent Progr Hormone Res*, 18:337, 1962.

FRAWLEY, T.F. Adrenal cortical insufficiency. *In* Eisenstein, A.B., ed. *The Adrenal Cortex*. Boston, Little, Brown and Co., 1967, Chap. 13.

GALLAGHER, T.F., FUKUSHIMA, D.K., NOGUCHI, S., FISHMAN, J., BRADLOW, H.L., CASSOUTO, J., ZUMOFF, D., and HELLMAN, L. Recent studies in steroid hormone metabolism in man. *Recent Progr Hormone Res*, 22:283, 1966.

LIDDLE, G.W. Cushing's syndrome. *In* Eisenstein, A.B., ed. *The Adrenal Cortex*. Boston, Little, Brown and Co., 1967, Chap. 14.

LISBOA, B.P., and DICZFALUSY, E. Separation and characterisation of steroid oestrogens by means of thin-layer chromatography. *Acta Endocr (Kobenhavn)*, 40:60, 1962.

MARGRAF, H.W., and WEICHSELBAUM, T.E. Laboratory procedures in diagnosis of adrenal cortical diseases. *In* Eisenstein, A.B., ed. *The Adrenal Cortex*. Boston, Little, Brown and Co., 1967, Chap. 12.

PORTER, C.C., and SILBER, R.H. A quantitative color reaction for corticosterone and related 17,21-dihydroxy-20-ketosteroids. *J Biol Chem*, 185:201, 1950.

ROSENFELD, R.S., FUKUSHIMA, D.K., and GALLAGHER, T.F. Metabolism of adrenal cortical hormones. *In* Eisenstein, A.B., ed. *The Adrenal Cortex*. Boston, Little, Brown and Co., 1967, Chap. 3.

SILBER, R.H., and PORTER, C.C. The determination of 17,21-dihydroxy-20-ketosteroids in urine and plasma. *J Biol Chem*, 210:923, 1954.

VANDE WIELE, R.L., MACDONALD, P.C., GURPIDE, E., and LIEBERMAN, S. Studies on the secretion and inter-conversion of the androgens. *Recent Progr Hormone Res*, 19:275, 1963.

9

Lipid Metabolism and Its Regulation

Lipids are a heterogeneous group of compounds that are extractable from living matter by organic solvents, but not by water. The classification scheme given in Table 1 was adapted from Cantarow and Schepartz.

Most of the lipid in animal adipose tissue (depot fat) is present in the form of triglyceride, for which a general formula is given in Figure 1.

Table 2 illustrates formulas for some common animal saturated and unsaturated fatty acids. Most of animal depot fat is composed of palmitic, stearic, and oleic acids. Human adipose, for example, contains larger percentages of oleic and palmitic acids, and smaller amounts of stearic, palmitoleic, linoleic, linolenic, and higher polyunsaturated fatty acids. Most other animal cells have fatty acids incorporated into phospholipid (see Figure 2 for some examples) and esterified to cholesterol, as shown in Figure 3.

LIPID FUNCTIONS

Physiologically the lipids provide a source and a storage form of energy, as well as a source of carbon, phosphorous, and nitrogen for metabolism. They func-

105

Table 1. CLASSIFICATION OF LIPIDS*

I. Simple Lipids

A. Neutral fats (glycerol esters of fatty acids)

B. Waxes (fatty acid esters of alcohols other than glycerol, including cholesterol esters)

II. Compound Lipids

A. Phospholipids (compounds containing phosphoric acid in linkage with fatty acids and alcohol)
    1. Lecithins
    2. Cephalins
       a. Ethanolamine type
       b. Serine type
    3. Phosphoinositides
    4. Plasmalogens
    5. Phosphatidic acids
    6. Sphingomyelins

B. Glycolipids (compounds containing carbohydrate and fatty acid, but not glycerol or phosphoric acid)
    1. Cerebrosides
    2. Gangliosides

C. Lipoproteins

III. Derived Lipids

A. Fatty acids

B. Alcohols
    1. Acyclic alcohols
    2. Carotenoid alcohols
    3. Sterols
    4. D vitamins
    5. Inositol

C. Hydrocarbons
    1. Aliphatic, saturated hydrocarbons
    2. Carotenoid hydrocarbons
    3. Squalene

IV. Substances Associated with Lipids in Nature

A. Tocopherols

B. K vitamins

C. Steroids

*Adapted from Cantarow and Schepartz, *Biochemistry*, 3rd ed., 1962. Courtesy of W.B. Saunders Co.

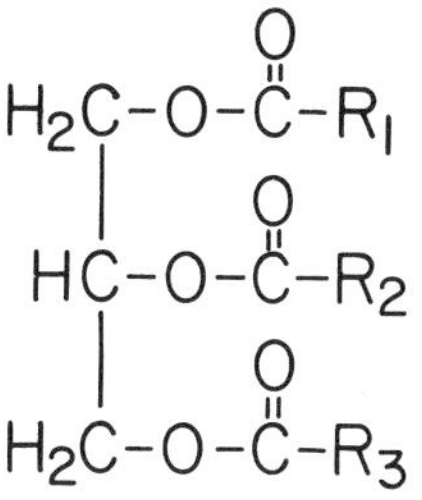

$$
\begin{array}{l}
\quad\quad\quad\quad\quad \overset{O}{\overset{\|}{}} \\
H_2C-O-C-R_1 \\
\quad\big| \quad\quad\overset{O}{\overset{\|}{}} \\
HC-O-C-R_2 \\
\quad\big| \quad\quad\overset{O}{\overset{\|}{}} \\
H_2C-O-C-R_3
\end{array}
$$

Fig. 1. Generic formula for the triglyceride structure. R-C(=O)- indicates the esterfied long-chain fatty acid, all three or only two of which may be different.

tion as detergent solubilizers for blood transport and digestion of hydrophobic substances. Lipids are also components of both basic types of mammalian membrane; the myelin membrane is composed of cholesterol, sphingolipid, and long-chain saturated fatty acids, while nuclear, mitochondrial, and microsomal membranes contain some sphingolipid or cholesterol and unsaturated phospho-

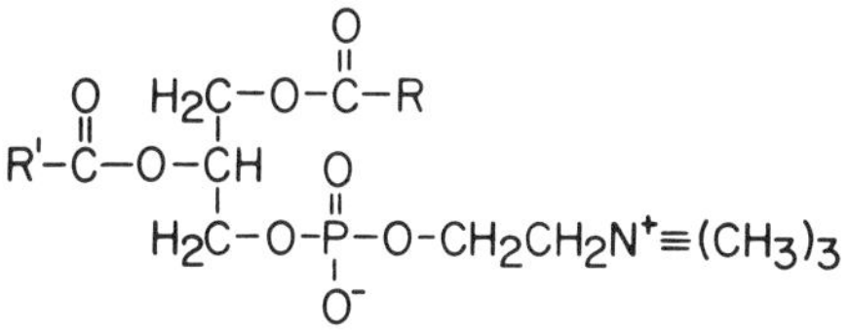

$$
\begin{array}{l}
\quad\quad\quad\quad\quad\quad \overset{O}{\overset{\|}{}} \\
\quad\quad O \quad H_2C-O-C-R \\
\quad\;\overset{\|}{} \quad\quad\big| \\
R'-C-O-CH \quad\; O \\
\quad\quad\quad\quad\big| \quad\;\;\overset{\|}{} \\
\quad\quad\; H_2C-O-P-O-CH_2CH_2N^+\equiv(CH_3)_3 \\
\quad\quad\quad\quad\quad\;\big| \\
\quad\quad\quad\quad\quad O^-
\end{array}
$$

LECITHIN

$$
\begin{array}{l}
\quad\quad\quad\quad\quad\quad \overset{O}{\overset{\|}{}} \\
\quad\quad O \quad H_2C-O-C-R \\
\quad\;\overset{\|}{} \quad\quad\big| \\
R'-C-O-CH \quad\; O \\
\quad\quad\quad\quad\big| \quad\;\;\overset{\|}{} \\
\quad\quad\; H_2C-O-P-O-CH_2CH_2\overset{+}{N}H_3 \\
\quad\quad\quad\quad\quad\;\big| \\
\quad\quad\quad\quad\quad O^-
\end{array}
$$

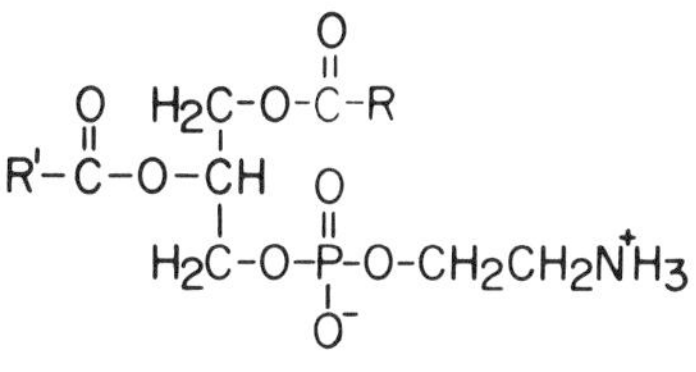

PHOSPHATIDYL ETHANOLAMINE

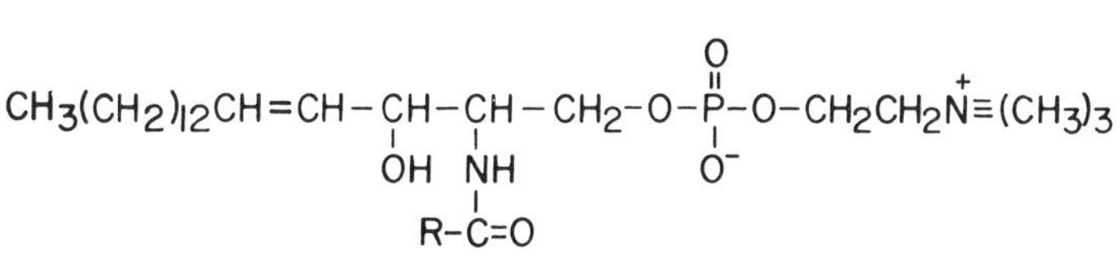

$$
CH_3(CH_2)_{12}CH=CH-CH-CH-CH_2-O-\overset{\overset{O}{\|}}{P}-O-CH_2CH_2\overset{+}{N}\equiv(CH_3)_3
$$
$$
\quad\quad\quad\quad\quad\quad\;\; OH \;\; NH \quad\quad\quad\; O^-
$$
$$
\quad\quad\quad\quad\quad\quad\quad\quad\;\; R-C=O
$$

SPHINGOMYELIN

Fig. 2. Some exemplary phospholipid compounds. R-C(=O)- indicates an esterified long-chain fatty acid, saturated or unsaturated.

Table 2. SOME COMMON FATTY ACIDS

Systematic Name	Common Name	Formula
Saturated		
n-Hexanoic	n-Butyric	$CH_3(CH_2)_2COOH$
n-Octanoic	Caproic	$CH_3(CH_2)_4COOH$
n-Decanoic	Caprylic	$CH_3(CH_2)_6COOH$
n-Dodecanoic	Capric	$CH_3(CH_2)_8COOH$
n-Tetradecanoic	Lauric	$CH_3(CH_2)_{10}COOH$
n-Hexadecanoic	Myristic	$CH_3(CH_2)_{12}COOH$
n-Octadecanoic	Palmitic	$CH_3(CH_2)_{14}COOH$
n-Eicosanoic	Stearic	$CH_3(CH_2)_{16}COOH$
	Arachidic	$CH_3(CH_2)_{18}COOH$
Unsaturated		
9-Hexadecenoic	Palmitoleic	$CH_3(CH_2)_5CH=CH(CH_2)_7COOH$
cis-9-Octadecenoic	Oleic	$CH_3(CH_2)_7CH=CH(CH_2)_7COOH$
11-Octadecenoic	Vaccenic	$CH_3(CH_2)_5CH=CH(CH_2)_9COOH$
cis,cis-9,12-Octadecadienoic	Linoleic	$CH_3(CH_2)_4CH=CHCH_2CH=CH(CH_2)_7COOH$
9,12,15-Octadecatrienoic	Linolenic	$CH_3CH_2CH=CHCH_2CH=CHCH_2CH=CH(CH_7)\ COOH$
5,8,11,14-Eicosatetraenoic	Arachidonic	$CH_3(CH_2)_4CH=CHCH_2CH=CHCH_2CH=CHCH_2CH=CH(CH_2)_3COOH$

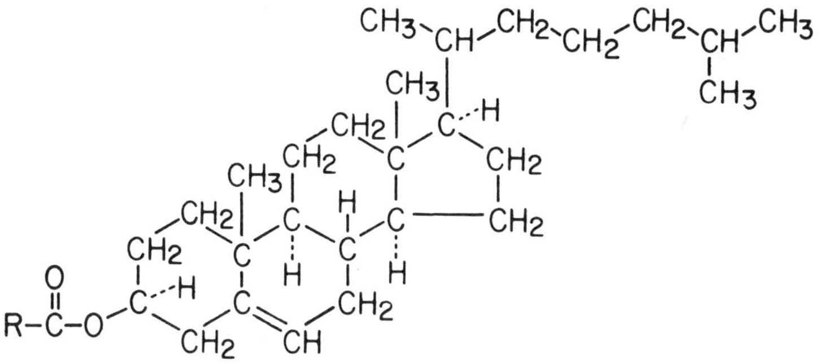

Fig. 3. Cholesterol esterified at the 3β-position with a long-chain fatty acid, e.g. palmitic acid (C16). The long-chain fatty acid is represented by R-C(=O)-.

lipids. In certain membranes, such as those of mitochondria, lipids as protein complexes are part of the solid state (nonaqueous) electron-transport system for ATP synthesis and other reactions such as steroid hydroxylation. Lipids have been recognized as covalently bound intermediates during condensation reactions in the biosynthesis of polysaccharides for the cell wall of some microorganisms. Phospholipids may also form activiating complexes with some enzymes and substrates.

DIGESTION AND ABSORPTION

Most dietary lipids reach the small intestine in the triglyceride form, where they are attacked by pancreatic lipase, which hydrolyzes medium- and long-chain fatty acids from the triglyceride in the presence of conjugated bile salts to give bile salt micelles of β-monoglycerides and free fatty acids. The micelles then are absorbed by the upper small intestine, and in the intestinal mucosa most of the absorbed monoglyceride is reacylated to triglyceride, although some is hydrolyzed and some converted to phospholipid. Reconstituted triglyceride is carried to the blood via the lymph for distribution to body tissues. Chylomicrons, small lipid particles surrounded by a protein coat, are the forms in which lipid travels in both blood and lymph. Any absorbed free fatty acids are transported by the portal system to the liver to be oxidized.

CELL COMPONENTS AND LIPID METABOLISM

Lipid metabolism occurs in many tissues of the body and is especially prominent in adipose tissue, mammary gland, liver, and endocrine tissues.

Several components of the cell contribute to lipid metabolism. The de novo fatty acid synthesis is accomplished by enzymes in the nonparticulate fraction of the cell, or cell supernatant. The mitochondrion is capable of activating fatty acids to their coenzyme A derivatives and elongating medium- and long-chain fatty acids. The mitochondrion is the sole site of fatty acid oxidation. It also demonstrates some phospholipase activity.

Microsomes, sedimented fragments of endoplasmic reticulum, can activate, elongate, and desaturate medium- or long-chain fatty acids to produce triglycerides, cholesterol esters, phospholipids, and glycolipids. They also have phospholipase activity and are the site for α and ω fatty acid oxidation. It is the smooth, not rough, endoplasmic reticulum that seems to be associated with lipid metabolism. Lysosomes appear to contain an active phospholipase.

A helpful table listing the intercellular distribution of enzymes of lipid metabolism has been formulated by Tubbs and Garland.

FATTY ACID BIOSYNTHETIC SYSTEMS

Four distinct systems for fatty acid synthesis appear to reside in animal tissue:

1. The first and best-studied mechanism is the fatty acid synthetase present in cell cytoplasm. It uses malonyl-CoA as the unit for condensation with acetyl-CoA and NADPH for the reductive steps in de novo synthesis.
2. Heart mitochondria, at least, appear to synthesize fatty acids by a reversal of β-oxidation using acetyl-CoA as the condensing unit and NADH for reducing equivalents.
3. Mitochondria also elongate preexisting fatty acids, employing acetyl-CoA and NADH.
4. The microsomes also have an elongation system which condenses malonyl-CoA with acyl-CoA and is characterized by showing no preference for either NADH or NADPH as a supplier of reducing power.

These systems will now be described in detail.

Fatty Acid Biosynthesis in the Cytoplasm

The cytoplasm is the site for the major portion of fatty acid synthesis; consequently this system is better defined than other systems as a result of intensive experimental investigation. The overall equation for the de novo biosynthesis of palmitic acid, a common end product of mammalian fatty acid synthesis, is shown in Figure 4. The intermediates of this reaction, which will be examined in detail, apparently are bound to a complex of six or seven enzymes which releases only the final product, palmitic acid. Eight molecules of the two-carbon unit, acetic acid, activated by their linkage to coenzyme A (see Fig. 5), are condensed. ATP supplies energy and two NADPH molecules donate the reducing equivalents for each of the condensations. Carbon dioxide is used and regenerated during the course of the reaction to provide the driving force for one of the intermediate steps.

A more detailed presentation of fatty acid biosynthesis is illustrated in Figure 6. By repeating the reactions given in equations 3 to 6 six more times, condensing malonyl-ACP with the product of equation 6, the carbon chain of the fatty acid will have grown to 16 carbons to form palmityl-ACP. A deacylase enzyme hydrates palmityl-ACP to palmitic acid and acyl carrier protein. This reaction is shown in equation 7. The lipogenesis sequence is catalyzed by a complex of six or seven enzymes called the fatty acid synthetase. Specific transacylases transfer the acetyl and malonyl moieties of acetyl-CoA and malonyl-CoA, respectively, to acyl carrier protein, forming acetyl-ACP and malonyl-ACP. These are condensed to yield acetoacetyl-ACP, while the concomitant decarboxylation insures a favorable equilibrium for the reaction. $NADPH + H^+$ reduces acetoacetyl-ACP to β-hydroxy-butyryl-ACP, which in turn is dehydrated to crotonyl-ACP. Butyryl-ACP is subsequently formed by $NADPH + H^+$ reduction of the crotonyl-ACP. By repetition of the cycle six times from the point where malonyl-ACP condenses with acyl-ACP, a molecule of palmityl-ACP is formed. The mammalian fatty acid synthetase generally terminates the synthesis at the 16-carbon-atom chain length, and a deacylase (palmityl thioesterase) hydrates palmityl-ACP to palmitic acid.

Sources of Carbon

As has been described in Figure 6, acetyl-CoA and malonyl-CoA provide the carbons for fatty acid synthesis. Acetyl-CoA, the primary carbon source for

$$8CH_3 - \overset{\overset{\displaystyle O}{\|}}{C} - SCoA + 7CO_2 + 7ATP + 14\ NADPH + 14H^+ \longrightarrow$$

$$CH_3(CH_2)_{14}COOH + 7CO_2 + 8CoASH + 7\ ADP + 7Pi + 14NADP^+ + 6H_2O$$

Fig. 4. Overall equation for the synthesis of palmitic acid that can occur de novo on the fatty acid synthetase complex in the cytoplasm of cells in tissues such as the liver and adipose tissue. Eight molecules of acetyl-CoA, 7 of carbon dioxide, 7 of adenosine triphosphate, and 14 reducing equivalents from NADPH, along with 14 hydrogen ions, are utilized in the formation of one molecule of palmitic acid.

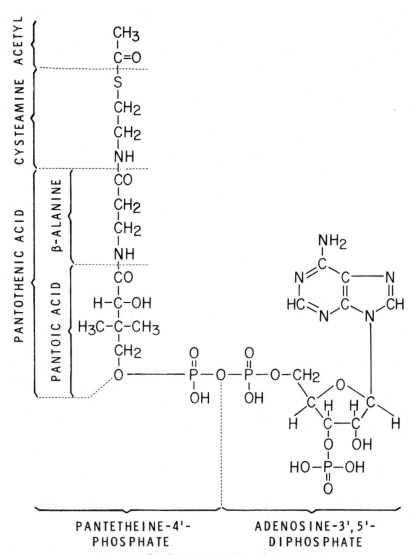

Fig. 5. Acetyl coenzyme A.

fatty acids, is formed intramitochondrially from the oxidation of pyruvate, the glycolytic product which readily enters the mitochondrion. The formation of pyruvate by glycolysis is described in Chapter 3, and the conversion of pyruvate to acetyl-CoA is illustrated in Figure 7. When glucose is adequate or in excess, pyruvate is derived largely from the metabolism of glucose-6-phosphate by glycolysis. Pyruvate can be converted to acetyl-CoA or oxalacetate. These compounds can condense to form citrate to be oxidized in the citric acid cycle.

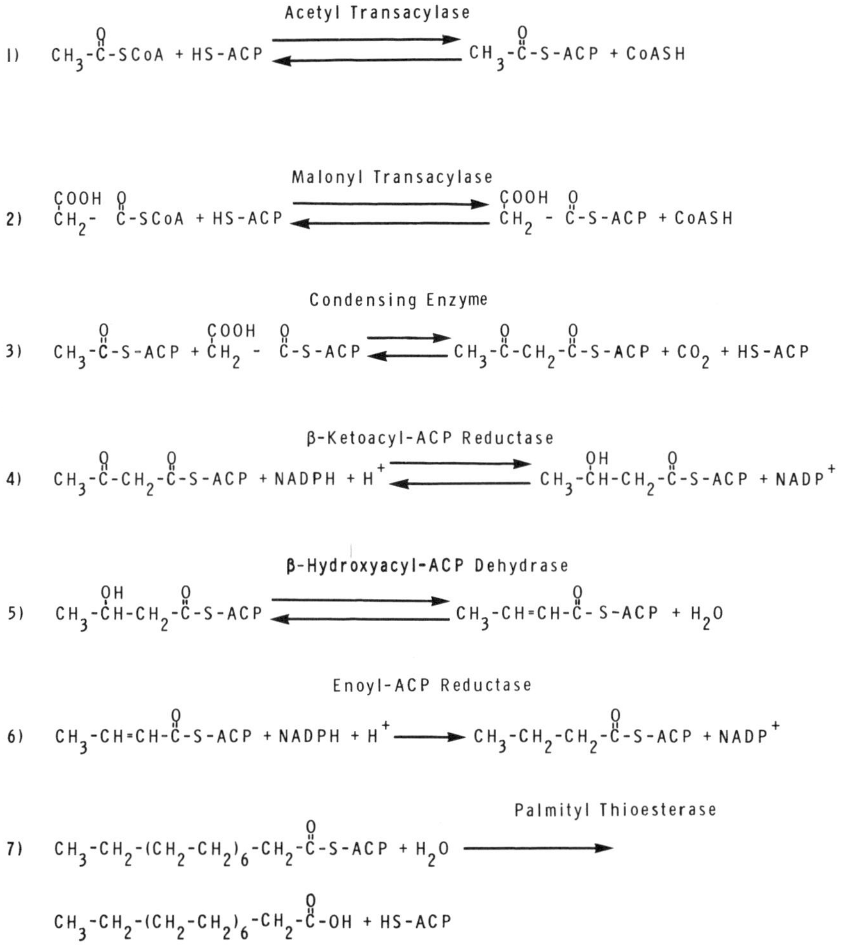

Acetyl Transacylase

1) $CH_3-\overset{O}{\overset{\|}{C}}-SCoA + HS-ACP \rightleftarrows CH_3-\overset{O}{\overset{\|}{C}}-S-ACP + CoASH$

Malonyl Transacylase

2) $\overset{COOH}{\underset{CH_2-}{|}} \overset{O}{\overset{\|}{C}}-SCoA + HS-ACP \rightleftarrows \overset{COOH}{\underset{CH_2}{|}} \overset{O}{\overset{\|}{C}}-S-ACP + CoASH$

Condensing Enzyme

3) $CH_3-\overset{O}{\overset{\|}{C}}-S-ACP + \overset{COOH}{\underset{CH_2}{|}} - \overset{O}{\overset{\|}{C}}-S-ACP \rightleftarrows CH_3-\overset{O}{\overset{\|}{C}}-CH_2-\overset{O}{\overset{\|}{C}}-S-ACP + CO_2 + HS-ACP$

β-Ketoacyl-ACP Reductase

4) $CH_3-\overset{O}{\overset{\|}{C}}-CH_2-\overset{O}{\overset{\|}{C}}-S-ACP + NADPH + H^+ \rightleftarrows CH_3-\overset{OH}{\underset{|}{C}}H-CH_2-\overset{O}{\overset{\|}{C}}-S-ACP + NADP^+$

β-Hydroxyacyl-ACP Dehydrase

5) $CH_3-\overset{OH}{\underset{|}{C}}H-CH_2-\overset{O}{\overset{\|}{C}}-S-ACP \rightleftarrows CH_3-CH=CH-\overset{O}{\overset{\|}{C}}-S-ACP + H_2O$

Enoyl-ACP Reductase

6) $CH_3-CH=CH-\overset{O}{\overset{\|}{C}}-S-ACP + NADPH + H^+ \longrightarrow CH_3-CH_2-CH_2-\overset{O}{\overset{\|}{C}}-S-ACP + NADP^+$

Palmityl Thioesterase

7) $CH_3-CH_2-(CH_2-CH_2)_6-CH_2-\overset{O}{\overset{\|}{C}}-S-ACP + H_2O \longrightarrow$

$CH_3-CH_2-(CH_2-CH_2)_6-CH_2-\overset{O}{\overset{\|}{C}}-OH + HS-ACP$

Fig. 6. Reactions in the synthesis of palmitic acid by a complex of six or seven enzymes called the fatty acid synthetase. In equation 1, the acetyl moiety of acetyl-CoA is transferred by acetyl transacylase to acyl carrier protein (ACP). A similar transfer of the malonyl moiety occurs as shown in equation 2. In equation 3, the condensing enzyme forms acetoacetyl-ACP with the release of carbon dioxide and one molecule of acyl carrier protein. In reaction 4, one reducing equivalent from NADPH is captured forming β-hydroxybutyryl-ACP. This compound is hydrated to crotonyl-ACP as shown in equation 5. In equation 6, another reducing equivalent is captured with the formation of butyryl-ACP. By repetition of the cycle six times beginning with the condensation reaction of equation 3, a molecule of palmityl-ACP is formed. A deacylase enzyme hydrates palmityl-ACP to palmitic acid and free acyl carrier protein.

Acetyl-CoA not required for energy production via the citric acid cycle is available for fatty acid and cholesterol synthesis and conversion to acetoacetate, the significance of which will be explained in connection with β-oxidation of fatty acids.

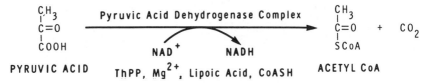

Fig. 7. The conversion of pyruvic acid to acetyl-CoA, catalyzed by the pyruvic acid dehydrogenase complex. The multienzyme complex found associated with mitochondria has been separated into components that catalyze the following reactions: 1. a magnesium-requiring decarboxylation of pyruvic acid and formation of enzyme-bound hydroxyethyl thiamine pyrophosphate by pyruvic acid decarboxylase bound with thiamine pyrophosphate (ThPP); 2. reduction of one of the thiol groups of enzyme-bound lipoic acid and transfer of the acetyl group to the other thiol of lipoic acid by the enzyme lipoic reductase-transacetylase; 3. transfer of the acetyl moiety to coenzyme A and consequent reduction of the lipoyl thiol to which the acetyl group was linked, a reaction catalyzed by the transacetylase; 4. oxidation of dihydrolipoate by dihydrogenase-bound FAD; and 5. a transhydrogenation transferring reducing equivalents from $FADH_2$ to NAD^+.

The mitochondrial membrane is impermeable to acetyl-CoA, creating the problem of transport of intramitochondrial acetyl-CoA into the cytoplasm for lipogenesis. There appear to be four possible solutions to the problem:

1. Some unknown mechanism for transport of acetyl-CoA directly across the membrane.
2. Cleavage of intramitochondrial acetyl-CoA, for which no adequate evidence has been presented, and transport of readily diffusible acetate across the membrane to the cytoplasm, where acetate thiokinase reforms acetyl-CoA.
3. Intramitochondrial formation of acetyl-carnitine, to which the membrane is permeable, and the cytoplasmic regeneration of acetyl-CoA, illustrated in Figure 8 and possibly forming a major mechanism for transport of acetyl-CoA out of the mitochondrion.
4. The citrate cleavage pathway, as shown in Figure 9 and as explained below.

The condensation of oxalacetate and acetyl-CoA in the mitochondrion as part of the citric acid cycle forms citrate, which can penetrate the mitochondrial

$$CH_3\text{-}\overset{O}{\overset{\|}{C}}\text{-SCoA} + (CH_3)_3\overset{+}{N}\text{-}CH_2\text{-}\underset{OH}{CH}\text{-}CH_2\text{-}COO^- \xrightleftharpoons \quad (CH_3)_3\overset{+}{N}\text{-}CH_2\text{-}\underset{O\text{-}\underset{O}{\overset{\|}{C}}\text{-}CH_3}{CH}\text{-}CH_2\text{-}COO^- + CoASH$$

Extramitochondrial

Intramitochondrial

Acetyl CoA   Carnitine   Acetyl Carnitine

Fig. 8. A mechanism for transport of acetyl-CoA out of the mitochondrion. Acetyl-CoA is formed by the oxidation of pyruvate in the mitochondria. Since the mitochondrial membrane is impermeable to acetyl-CoA, the acetyl group is transferred outside as acetyl-carnitine formed from a reaction catalyzed by intramitochondrial carnitine-acetyl transferase. Acetyl-CoA is regenerated on the cytoplasmic side of the mitochondrial membrane by the enzyme carnitine-acetyl transferase in the presence of extramitochondrial coenzyme A.

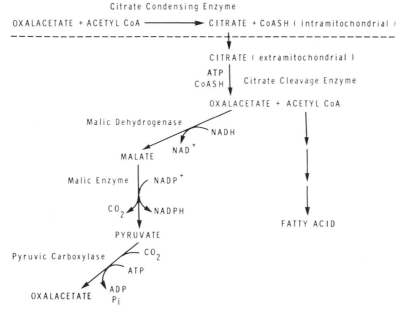

Fig. 9. A diagram illustrating various aspects of the citrate cleavage system which facilitates the transport of acetyl-CoA out of the mitochondrion and provides reducing equivalents for fatty acid synthesis. The condensation of oxalacetate and acetyl-CoA occurs as the initial reaction of the citric acid cycle in the mitochondrion. Citrate has the option of remaining in the mitochondrion for further oxidation in the cycle, or it may cross the mitochondrial membrane and be cleaved to oxalacetate and acetate by the citrate cleavage enzyme in the cytoplasm. After the cytoplasmic acetate is esterified to coenzyme A by acetate thiokinase, it is available to the fatty acid synthetase. Oxalacetate may be reduced by the extramitochondrial NAD^+-malic dehydrogenase to malate, and malate subsequently decarboxylated and oxidized to pyruvate by $NADP^+$-malic enzyme. This substrate-mediated transhydrogenation may well provide a portion of the NADPH used in fatty acid synthesis. Pyruvate can enter the mitochondrion and replenish oxalacetate of the citric acid cycle through the reaction catalyzed by pyruvic carboxylase.

membrane to the cytoplasm where the citrate cleavage enzyme catalyzes the formation of oxalacetate and acetyl-CoA. The oxalacetate is reduced by extramitochondrial malic dehydrogenase and NADH to malate, which in turn is converted to pyruvate by a process of oxidation and decarboxylation, catalyzed by the $NADP^+$-coupled malic enzyme. Thus, extramitochondrial NADPH for fatty acid synthesis can be provided. Oxalacetate can be resupplied to the intramitochondrial citric acid cycle by pyruvate carboxylase which utilizes pyruvate and CO_2 as shown in Figure 10. The citrate cleavage pathway may be a major regulator of fatty acid synthesis by providing most of the extramitochondrial acetyl-CoA. It appears that the citrate cleavage enzyme increases secondarily to increased lipogenesis to sustain an adequate supply of acetyl CoA (Foster and Srere).

Malonyl CoA is a product of acetyl CoA by a reaction catalyzed by acetyl-CoA carboxylase whose activity correlates with variations in synthetase

Pyruvate Carboxylase

$$Pyruvate + CO_2 + ATP \xrightarrow{\hspace{5cm}} Oxalacetate + ADP + Pi$$

Enzyme-Bound Biotin
Acetyl CoA
Mg^{2+} or Mn^{2+}

Fig. 10. The formation of oxalacetate from pyruvate by the pyruvate carboxylase reaction. The enzyme contains biotin as a prosthetic group and absolutely requires acetyl-CoA as a cofactor which may act by maintaining an active conformation of the enzyme. The divalent cations are also needed as cofactors. Energy for this CO_2 fixation reaction is supplied by ATP hydrolysis.

activities (Chang et al.). This implies that the activity of the carboxylase is not rate-limiting to fatty acid synthesis. Acetyl-CoA carboxylase catalyzes the carboxylation of acetyl-CoA to malonyl-CoA and requires ATP and biotin, as shown in Figure 11. The enzyme appears to be conformationally activated by polycarboxylic acids, especially citric and isocitric acids, and by bovine serum albumin, all of which may act by chelating metallosalts of fatty acids which can prevent trimerization of the carboxylase. The enzyme is inhibited by malonyl-CoA as well as by long-chain fatty acyl-CoA's, an example of a feedback inhibition mechanism. Acetyl-CoA carboxylase is associated with the microsomal membrane but is released to the cytoplasm in the absence of Mg^{++}.

Sources of Reductive Hydrogen

Reducing equivalents for cytoplasmic fatty acid synthesis are supplied by reduced $NADP^+$. The four $NADP^+$-coupled dehydrogenases of the cytoplasm—glucose-6-phosphate dehydrogenase, 6-phosphogluconate dehydrogenase, isocitric dehydrogenase, and malic enzyme—have been considered as sources for this reductive hydrogen. Reactions for glucose-6-phosphate dehydrogenase and 6-phosphogluconate dehydrogenase are given in Chapter 2, while $NADP^+$-malic enzyme is discussed in Figure 8 of Chapter 3. Various studies have determined that the two pentose cycle dehydrogenases, glucose-6-phosphate dehydrogenase

Acetyl CoA Carboxylase

$$CH_3\overset{O}{\overset{\|}{C}}\text{-SCoA} + ATP + CO_2 \underset{\longleftarrow}{\overset{\longrightarrow}{\hspace{3cm}}} \overset{COOH}{\underset{CH_2}{}} - \overset{O}{\overset{\|}{C}}\text{-SCoA} + ADP + Pi$$

Mg^{2+} or Mn^{2+}

Biotin (attached covalently
to the enzyme)

Fig. 11. The formation of malonyl-CoA from acetyl-CoA and carbon dioxide, with ATP energy enzyme acetyl-CoA carboxylase, which contains covalently bound biotin.

(G-6-PD) and 6-phosphogluconate dehydrogenase (6-PGD), the $NADP^+$-malic enzyme, and NAD^+-malic dehydrogenase, which forms a transhydrogenation system with $NADP^+$-malic enzyme, exhibit variations in activity in accord with nutritionally and hormonally induced fluctuations in lipogenesis. Isocitric dehydrogenase does not show these same variations. It has also been noted that the distribution of the pentose phosphate cycle dehydrogenases and of malic enzyme in various rat tissues is directly related to the capacity of the tissue for fatty acid synthesis. The pentose phosphate cycle is discussed in Chapter 2.

Studies of the fatty acid synthesizing system of the mammary gland showed that the efficiency of tritium transfer to fatty acids from the α position on C-4 of NADPH was greater than from the β position. Since the pentose cycle dehydrogenases are specific for the β position and isocitric dehydrogenase for the α, it would be expected that glucose-6-phosphate and 6-phosphogluconate are unfavorable substrates for producing NADPH for fatty acid synthesis, whereas isocitrate would be a favorable substrate (Matthes et al.). But in rat liver the isocitric dehydrogenase does not appear to be closely associated with lipogenesis, while the other $NADP^+$-dehydrogenases do. Perhaps by virtue of the high turnover rate in liver, NADPH randomizes more quickly than fatty acids are synthesized, allowing the pentose phosphate cycle dehydrogenases to supply reducing equivalents for lipogenesis.

Although experimental evidence indicates that the quantity of NADPH formed via the pentose cycle in adipose tissue is sufficient for only 50 to 65 percent of all of the fatty acid synthesis from glucose during conditions of rapid lipogenesis, the NADPH thus formed is tightly coupled to the fatty acid synthesis. The quantity of NADH produced by glycolysis in adipose is far in excess of that required for production of glycerol phosphate from dihydroxyace-tone phosphate and for conversion of pyruvate to lactate. Thus, it has been postulated that substrate mediated transhydrogenation of the excess of NADH by NAD^+-coupled malic dehydrogenase and $NADP^+$-coupled malic enzyme of the citrate cleavage system (Fig. 9) can supply about 35 percent of NADPH needed for fatty acid biosynthesis from glucose. The remaining approximately one half of the NADH is reoxidized via oxidative phosphorylation. Since in the electron-transport sequence for the synthesis of ATP, oxygen is consumed, the oxidation of the NADH may explain the 72 percent increase in oxygen consumption found during increased conversion of glucose to fatty acid that is induced by insulin. At the same time, NADH from increased glycolysis may replace NADH generated from the citric acid cycle as an energy source, and the citric acid cycle may shut down. Thus, more acetyl-CoA will be channeled into fatty acid, providing a greater efficiency for lipogenesis (Flatt and Ball).

The rate of reduction of $NADP^+$ by the pentose phosphate cycle could regulate fatty acid synthesis. On the other hand, it is possible that the rate of utilization of NADPH regulates the pentose phosphate cycle. In support of the latter idea, Flatt and Ball showed that the addition of acetate to a system in which glucose is converted to fatty acids increases the activity of the pentose cycle by 83 percent. It has been found, also, that glucose induced, in livers of newly hatched chicks or of rats, an increase in lipogenesis which was not dependent on an immediately concomitant increase in the activity of malic or citrate cleavage enzymes (Goodridge; Foster and Srere). Perhaps the increased consumption of NADPH was provided for by increased pentose phosphate cycle activity. However, other studies of rat liver and adipose showed that enhanced lipogenesis was accompanied by increased activity of both malic and citrate cleavage enzymes (Ball).

In summary, it must be stated that apparently no single mechanism supplies either all the carbon or all the reducing equivalents for fatty acid biosynthesis. Certainly the acetyl-CoA formed from pyruvate in the mitochondrion is the primary carbon source for fatty acid synthesis, but exactly how the acetyl-CoA is transported through the mitochondrial membrane to the cytoplasm remains uncertain. The two most likely possibilities for the transport are the acyl-carnitine and citrate cleavage systems.

Some uncertainty also prevails in connection with the primary source of reductive hydrogen in the form of NADPH for cytoplasmic fatty acid synthesis. Probably both the pentose phosphate cycle and substrate-mediated transhydrogenation contribute to the supply of NADPH for synthesis, but the relative importance of each at any given time may vary as a result of metabolic and experimental conditions. The citrate cleavage system alone may provide both a transport mechanism for acetyl-CoA and a source of reducing equivalents through the malic dehydrogenase and the malic enzyme.

Fatty Acid Synthetases of the Cytoplasm

The fatty acid synthetases isolated from the cytoplasm of mammalian liver, brain, mammary gland, and adipose and from the cytoplasm of yeast and of pigeon liver have not been resolved into their components. However, the synthetase complexes of E. coli, Clostridium sp., and various plants, such as avocado mesocarp, and lettuce and spinach chloroplasts, are readily dissociated into two or more parts. For example, the extensively studied E. coli synthetase has yielded upon dissociation six enzymes concerned in fatty acid synthesis— acetyl transacylase, malonyl transacylase, condensing enzyme, β-ketoacyl-ACP reductase, enoyl-ACP hydrase, and crotonyl-ACP reductase. The seventh enzyme, the deacylase, may or may not be associated with the synthetase complex itself. The different synthetases isolated from various species differ to some extent in composition and structure. For instance, yeast fatty acid synthetase requires flavin mononucleotide as a cofactor and has a molecular weight of 2.3×10^6, while pigeon liver synthetase requires no flavin coenzyme and has a molecular weight estimated at 5.4×10^5. All the cytoplasmic synthetases may differ slightly with respect to chain length of the fatty acids they generate. The final fatty acid synthesized may be bound to coenzymes A, as with the yeast complex, or unbound as free fatty acid in the case of mammalian systems.

One component that the dissociable synthetases have in common is the heat-stable protein of low molecular weight, the acyl carrier protein (ACP). Indirect evidence indicates that ACP is also involved in the undissociable synthetase complexes. A comparative study of two purified bacterial and two purified plant ACP's revealed a similarity of amino acid composition and molecular weight in all four. Between the two sets, the most significant difference was a greater lysine content of the plant ACP's. Cross-reacting the bacterial and plant ACP's with a plant or bacterial synthetase yields different fatty acids from the usual product of each synthetase system.

Lynen's concept of the structure of his fatty acid synthetase, purified from yeast, is that of a complex of six constituent enzymes arranged sequentially around a central core which may be the acyl carrier protein. The intermediates of fatty acid synthesis, covalently bound to the thiol group of the ACP, can rotate with it, thus bringing the intermediates into contact with each of the enzymes in turn. A "peripheral" thiol group has been associated with the condensing enzyme of the complex and may be instrumental in determining the specificity of the complex in terminating fatty acid synthesis at the 16th or 18th carbon in the chain (Lynen). The length of the carbon chain of the bound fatty acid may also determine the cutoff point of de novo synthesis and release of the fatty acid from the synthetase, simply by the increasing instability of the bond between the fatty acid and the protein enzyme complex.

Fatty Acid Synthesis in the Mitochondria

The mitochondrion contains a system for chain elongation of preexisting saturated and unsaturated fatty acids as their coenzyme A derivatives. The condensing unit for chain elongation of the fatty acyl-CoA appears to be malonyl CoA and the reducing equivalents may be supplied by NADPH. The mechanism for chain elongation is essentially that of reactions 3-6 shown in Figure 6 but starting with fatty acyl-CoA ($CH_3(CH_2)_n$-(C=O)-SCoA) instead of acetyl-ACP (CH_3-(C=O)-S-ACP). In every case derivatives are with CoA instead of ACP. Earlier research has suggested the existence of a de novo system very similar to the cytoplasmic system, starting from acetyl CoA and using malonyl CoA as its condensing unit (Harlin and Wakil). However, this finding may have been due to contamination of the mitochondrial preparation with cytoplasmic synthetase. Recent studies of Wakil and coworkers have demonstrated that mitochondria are not capable of de novo synthesis of fatty acids from acetyl CoA, using malonyl CoA as the condensing unit.

Recently, it has been suggested (Whereat et al.; Christ) that heart mitochondria at least, can synthesize fatty acids by a reversal of the β-oxidation system, which will be described later, utilizing acetyl CoA as the condensing unit. The regulation of the operational direction of the system may lie in the NADH: NAD^+ ratio of the mitochondria. If a correct hypothesis, this fatty acid oxidation-synthesis cycle has important implications for the energy metabolism of the cell. It is known that the heart derives most of its energy requirement from the oxidation of fatty acids. The oxidation of fatty acids to acetyl-CoA and of acetyl-CoA to carbon dioxide occurs when there is a requirement for energy in the form of ATP generated by oxidative phosphorylation in the electron-transport chain. There must be abundant ADP as the phosphate acceptor and available oxygen to capture reducing equivalents for the electron-transport chain to operate. If either phosphate acceptor or oxygen is unavailable or limited, then lipogenesis occurs even in the presence of an adequate supply of fatty acids. Thus the cycle could provide a storage system for the energy to be derived from acetate and NADH, as well as a mechanism for the oxidation of NADH when oxygen is unavailable, as in the physiologic state of oxygen debt (Whereat et al.).

Fatty Acid Synthesis in the Microsomes

Microsomes present a fourth distinct system for lipogenesis. They do not synthesize fatty acids de novo, but do elongate 10 carbon (10C) or longer fatty acyl-CoA's, using malonyl-CoA as the condensing unit. Only when a double bond is present will microsomes elongate a fatty acyl-CoA longer than 16C. The main products of rat and pigeon liver microsomal systems are saturated and unsaturated 18C and 20C fatty acids incorporated into phospholipids and cholesterol esters.

Although the microsomal system requires reduced pyridine nucleotide for synthesis, it appears to have no specificity for either NADH or NADPH, which may imply that the microsomal fatty acids are important for storage of reducing equivalents from NAD^+-coupled reactions as well as from the $NADP^+$ dehydrogenases. ATP is a required compound also, probably for activating long-chain fatty acids to fatty acyl-CoA, and for synthesizing phospholipids. The microsomal system reacts most readily with saturated and polyunsatured 10C to 16C acyl-CoA's. Chain elongation occurs by the same four reactions described for mitochondrial elongation of fatty acids. The intermediates are CoA derivatives, rather than bound to ACP as they are with the cytoplasmic synthetase.

Fatty Acid Desaturation

The fatty acid desaturase systems operate either aerobically or anaerobically, depending on the oxygen requirement of the organisms to which they belong. For the most part, these systems are present in the microsomal cell fraction, and the enzymes appear to be localized on the membrane of the endoplasmic reticulum rather than on the ribosomes. There may be a soluble desaturase system in some plants and bacteria.

The anaerobic desaturation of fatty acids present in anaerobic bacteria such as *E. coli* is closely associated with the de novo synthesis of saturated fatty acids in the same organism. When the growing fatty acid has reached a medium chain length of 10C to 12C, a dehydrase removes water from β-hydroxyacyl-ACP and introduces a double bond at the β-γ position instead of the α-β position as in saturated fatty acid synthesis. The double bond is not reduced via NADPH, but is left in position while the chain further elongates normally to a 16C or 18C fatty acid, yielding palmitoleic or *cis*-vaccenic acids as the unsaturated fatty acids of *E. coli*.

The aerobic system of yeast and animals requires molecular oxygen, reduced pyridine nucleotide, and a monooxygenase. The mechanism for the reaction has yet to be elucidated but it may involve the same cytochrome c reductase and cytochrome P_{450} system that catalyzes steroid hydroxylations. It is known that stearyl-CoA or stearyl-ACP is the predominate substrate for the desaturase of rat liver which produces oleic acid. The animal organ that contributes most to elongation and desaturation of fatty acids is the liver.

The synthesis of polyunsaturated fatty acids of animal tissue usually follows a pattern of desaturation, then a two-carbon elongation, followed by a number of repetitions of the pattern. There is some evidence that the metabolism of some animals, including humans, does not provide a sufficient supply of these polyunsaturated fatty acids; consequently linoleic, linolenic, and arachidonic acids may be considered essential to the diet.

Hydrogenation of unsaturated fatty acids is of little consequence in animals, although it may be important in some microorganisms.

FATTY ACID CATABOLISM

The pathways to be discussed are those participating in the degradation of fatty acids in animal, especially mammalian, tissue. Plants and microorganisms may exhibit modified routes of fatty acid breakdown.

Beta Oxidation in the Mitochondria

By far the most prevalent pathway for fatty acid degradation is the β-oxidation enzyme system which catalyzes the stepwise cleavage of two-carbon units from the long-chain fatty acyl-CoA beginning from the carboxyl end. This β-oxidation system resides in the mitochondrion and uses NAD^+ and FAD as acceptors of the reducing equivalents, which eventually provide the usable form of energy derived from fatty acid oxidation. Some studies even imply that the β-oxidation system may exist as a multienzyme complex (Tubbs and Garland). For the most part, the cleavage process proceeds directly to acetyl-CoA without interruption, leaving no free fatty acids of medium chain length to be detected as intermediates of the reaction.

A summary equation for fatty acid oxidation is exemplified by the equation for the oxidation of palmitic acid, as illustrated in Figure 12. In order for fatty acid oxidation to commence, some polycarboxylic acids of the citric acid cycle must be present in catalytic amounts for three reasons. They must be available to provide the energy of ATP (derived from reoxidation of reduced coenzymes generated through operation of the citric acid cycle) for activation of fatty acids to acyl-CoA's. The polycarboxylic acids also provide the oxalacetate (via the citric acid cycle) which must condense with acetyl-CoA generated from fatty acid oxidation so that complete oxidation of the fatty acid might occur. Oxalacetate may also be provided by the pyruvate carboxylase reaction. The condensation of acetyl-CoA and oxalacetate also regenerates coenzyme A for further fatty acid activation, thus revealing a third purpose of this "sparking" reaction by polycarboxylic acids.

The individual reactions of the β-oxidation scheme are illustrated in Figure 13. In the first reaction a fatty acid in the animal mitochondrion is activated to the fatty acyl-CoA by any one of the following enzymes: a medium-chain fatty acid thiokinase, a long-chain fatty acid thiokinase, or a thiophorase which catalyzes the transfer of the coenzyme from an acyl-CoA to a free fatty acid. The hydrolysis of ATP to AMP and pyrophosphate supplies the energy for this reaction.

If the fatty acyl-CoA resides outside the mitochondrion, a mechanism for transporting it across the mitochondrial membrane must be available, since fatty acyl-CoA, like acetyl-CoA, is unable to penetrate the membrane. The carnitine-acyl transferase reaction, similar to the one given previously for acetyl-CoA in Figure 8, could provide the necessary means for the transport and regeneration

$$CH_3(CH_2CH_2)_7COOH + ATP + 8CoASH + 7NAD^+ + 7FAD + 7H_2O \longrightarrow$$

$$8CH_3\overset{O}{\underset{}{C}}-SCoA + AMP + PPi + 7NADH + 7H^+ + 7FADH_2$$

Fig. 12. Summary equation for the oxidation of palmitic acid by β-oxidation. Both nicotinamide adenine dinucleotide (NAD^+) and flavin adenine dinucleotide (FAD) are hydrogen acceptors in the various reactions given in detail in the next figure.

Fatty Acid Thiokinase

(1) $R-CH_2CH_2COOH + ATP + CoASH \xrightleftharpoons{Mg^{2+}} R-CH_2CH_2-\overset{O}{\overset{\|}{C}}-SCoA + AMP + PPi$

Fatty Acyl CoA Dehydrogenase

(2) $R-CH_2CH_2-\overset{O}{\overset{\|}{C}}-SCoA + FAD \rightleftharpoons R-\overset{H}{\underset{H}{C}}-\overset{H}{C}-\overset{O}{\overset{\|}{C}}-SCoA + FADH_2$

Enoyl Hydrase

(3) $R-\overset{H}{\underset{H}{C}} = \overset{}{C}-\overset{O}{\overset{\|}{C}}-SCoA + H_2O \rightleftharpoons R-\overset{OH}{\underset{H}{C}}-CH_2-\overset{O}{\overset{\|}{C}}-SCoA$

β-Hydroxyacyl CoA Dehydrogenase

(4) $R-\overset{OH}{\underset{H}{C}}-CH_2-\overset{O}{\overset{\|}{C}}-SCoA + NAD^+ \rightleftharpoons R-\overset{O}{\overset{\|}{C}}-CH_2-\overset{O}{\overset{\|}{C}}-SCoA + NADH + H^+$

β-Ketothiolase

(5) $R-\overset{O}{\overset{\|}{C}}-CH_2-\overset{O}{\overset{\|}{C}}-SCoA + CoASH \rightleftharpoons R-\overset{O}{\overset{\|}{C}}-SCoA + CH_3-\overset{O}{\overset{\|}{C}}-SCoA$

Fig. 13. Beta-oxidation of fatty acids. The first reaction is activation of a free fatty acid to its coenzyme A ester by a thiokinase enzyme. ATP hydrolysis supplies the energy for this activation reaction. The fatty acyl-CoA must be transported across the mitochondrial membrane for catabolism inside the mitochondrion. Transport is probably accomplished by the reaction catalyzed by carnitine-acyl transferase, which resembles the carnitine-acetyl transferase reaction described previously. The second equation, but first reaction of the repeating set of reactions (2-5), shows the capturing of reducing equivalents by FAD with the formation of an α,β-unsaturated fatty acyl-CoA. The enzyme may be one of four fatty acyl-CoA dehydrogenases specific for certain chain lengths of fatty acids. In the reaction numbered 3, enoyl hydrase catalyzes the formation of an L-β-hydroxyacyl-CoA. In the next reaction, NAD$^+$ is reduced with the formation of a β-ketoacyl-CoA by the enzyme β-ketoacyl-CoA dehydrogenase, which is nonspecific in regard to fatty acid chain length. In reaction 5, a series of β-ketothiolases cleave acetyl-CoA from a corresponding series of chain lengths of β-ketoacyl-CoA compounds. The remaining product is activated with coenzyme A. The molecules of acetyl-CoA formed by this set of reactions are metabolized in the citric acid cycle by condensing with oxalacetate, and under normal circumstances, a small portion is converted to ketone bodies. Acetyl-CoA also normally serves as a cholesterol precursor.

Thus, in mitochondrial oxidation of fatty acids, hydrogen and an electron pair are captured by the electron carriers FAD and NAD$^+$. Part of the energy residing in the reduced coenzymes is captured in forming the high-energy compound ATP during passage of the reducing equivalents through the electron-transport sequence of the mitochondria for reoxidation. These metabolic sequences are given in Figure 9, Chapter 2.

of the coenzyme A derivative. This system will be examined in more detail as a control mechanism in a later section.

The second step of fatty acid oxidation, and first step of the repeating set of reactions, is catalyzed by one of four different fatty acyl-CoA dehydrogenases in mammalian liver mitochondria. They differ with respect to their specificities for certain chain lengths of fatty acids, but all four dehydrogenases use FAD as the coenzyme for capturing the reducing equivalents removed to form the α-β unsaturated fatty acyl-CoA.

The enoyl hydrase catalyzes the specific formation of L-β-hydroxyacyl-CoA from the trans-2-enoyl-CoA. The β-hydroxyacyl-CoA dehydrogenase requires NAD^+ as its coenzyme and is nonspecific with regard to chain length in converting its substrate to β-ketoacyl-CoA. In contrast, several β-ketothiolases may be necessary in a cell to cleave acetyl-CoA from all the β-ketoacyl compounds and to activate the remaining product with coenzyme A, since the isolated enzymes have been found to be specific for varying chain lengths. The set of reactions for equations 2 to 5 in Figure 13 repeats itself until only an acetyl-CoA remains after cleaving off acetyl-CoA from a four-carbon fatty acyl-CoA.

Fatty acid oxidation in the mitochondria is useful in providing for reduction of FAD and NAD^+ which, when reoxidized by the electron-transport chain, transfers energy to ATP needed for numerous energy-requiring cellular processes. Each two-carbon unit cleaved from a long-chain fatty acid by β-oxidation leads to the reduction of one FAD and one NAD^+; and oxidation of the acetyl-CoA via the citric acid cycle results in the reduction of one more FAD and three more NAD^+'s. Remembering that oxidation of $FADH_2$ by the oxidative phosphorylation process yields two ATP molecules, that oxidation of $NADH + H^+$ yields three ATP's, and that the citric acid cycle generates GTP which can transfer its high-energy phosphate to ATP, it can be calculated that for each two-carbon unit released and completely oxidized from a fatty acid longer than four carbons, 17 molecules of ATP are generated. The complete oxidation of one molecule of palmityl-CoA should yield 131 molecules of ATP.

There is no evidence to indicate that fatty acid oxidation in endocrine tissues that secrete steroids couples to the electron-transport sequence for steroid hydroxylation in the mitochondrion.

Odd-numbered fatty acids yield, upon conventional β-oxidation, a number of acetyl-CoA's and one molecule of propionyl-CoA. Mammalian metabolism of this propionyl-CoA, for the most part, proceeds on to succinyl-CoA by the reactions shown in Figure 14. There exist other routes of propionate metabolism, besides the one given above, in mammals, plants, and microorganisms.

Mitochondria are also capable of completely oxidizing polyunsaturated fatty acids by a β-oxidation mechanism which requires three additional enzymes—an isomerase, a hydrase, and an epimerase.

A portion of the acetyl-CoA pool in liver undergoes a condensation reaction which is the reverse of the thiolase reaction in β-oxidation. The major fate of the condensation product, acetoacetyl-CoA, is its conversion to an intermediate for cholesterol synthesis, β-hydroxy-β-methylglutaryl-CoA, through condensation with another molecule of acetyl-CoA. However, some of the β-hydroxy-β-methylglutaryl-CoA is normally degraded to acetoacetate and

(I)   Propionyl CoA + ATP + CO_2 $\underset{\substack{Mg^{2+} \\ Biotin}}{\overset{Carboxylase}{\rightleftharpoons}}$ S-Methylmalonyl CoA + ADP + Pi

(2)   S-Methylmalonyl CoA $\overset{Racemase}{\rightleftharpoons}$ R-Methylmalonyl CoA

(3)   R-Methylmalonyl CoA $\underset{B_{12}\ Coenzyme}{\overset{Mutase}{\rightleftharpoons}}$ Succinyl CoA

Fig. 14. Metabolism of propionyl-CoA. Oxidation of odd-numbered fatty acids by β-oxidation yields acetyl-CoA molecules and one molecule of propionyl-CoA. This is usually metabolized, as shown, to succinyl-CoA, which is a substrate of the citric acid cycle.

acetyl-CoA. The pools of both these acetate derivatives may be partly supplied through transformations of the ketogenic amino acids.

Acetoacetate is known as the primary ketone body, one of a group of compounds which accumulate in abnormally high levels under certain conditions when metabolic use of glucose is impaired. The ketone bodies include acetoacetate, β-hydroxybutyrate, and acetone. Acetoacetate is reduced by a DPN^+-dehydrogenase to form β-hydroxybutyrate, apparently when there is an adequate supply of DPNH available from metabolism. On the other hand, acetoacetate may undergo decarboxylation in the blood, possibly nonenzymatically, producing acetone. All three of the ketone bodies can be utilized by some tissues. Acetoacetate and β-hydroxybutyrate, reoxidized to acetoacetate, can be esterified to acetoacetyl-CoA and then cleaved to yield two molecules of acetyl-CoA. Acetone may be cleaved to acetyl and formyl fragments, or it can be transformed to pyruvic acid.

Under conditions that produce an abnormally large pool of acetyl-CoA, such as the high rate of fatty acid oxidation brought about during starvation or diabetes when glucose is not available to metabolism, abnormally high concentrations of ketone bodies appear in the circulation. To be more precise, Krebs postulates that the lack of oxalacetate, which has been diverted into gluconeogenesis, is a direct cause of ketosis. The decreased condensation of acetyl-CoA and oxalacetate diverts acetyl-CoA to ketone bodies such as acetoacetate. The danger of ketosis—a condition characterized by ketonemia, ketonuria, and acetone odor of the breath—lies in the acidosis and severe dehydration it causes if the condition goes unchecked.

Alpha and Omega Oxidation in the Microsomes

Two additional pathways of fatty acid oxidation have been located in the microsomes of mammalian tissue. Alpha oxidation occurs in brain microsomes and in some plants with a slightly altered pathway, and omega oxidation has been described in liver microsomes as well as in the supernatant of some bacterial cells.

Alpha oxidation provides a means for shortening long-chain fatty acids by one-carbon units. First, the fatty acid is oxidized to an α-hydroxy acid, probably by a monooxygenase using oxygen and $DMPH_2$ (6,7-dimethyl-5,6,7,8-tetra-hydropterin). The hydroxy acid is further oxidized by a NAD^+-dehydrogenase to an α-keto acid, which subsequently undergoes oxidative decarboxylation catalyzed by an enzyme which requires NAD^+, ATP, and ascorbic acid. The product is a fatty acid one carbon shorter than the original reactant.

Omega oxidation involves hydroxylation of a long-chain or, preferably, medium-chain fatty acid at the ω carbon, the end carbon opposite the carboxyl carbon. A monooxygenase catalyzes the reaction using molecular oxygen and NADPH, probably through the same enzyme system that hydroxylates the steroid hormones—namely, the NADPH-cytochrome reductase, cytochrome P_{450} system (Das et al.). The ω-hydroxylated acid is oxidized again to give the medium- or long-chain dicarboxylic acid, which may then be degraded via β-oxidation from either end, or it may be excreted directly.

TRIGLYCERIDE METABOLISM

Triglyceride is the predominant form of fat stored in adipose tissue for use as an energy source. It is also the most prevalent form in which fatty acids are incorporated in chylomicrons for transport in the lymph and blood to various parts of the body.

Triglyceride Synthesis

L-α-Glycerophosphate is a prerequisite for triglyceride biosynthesis, and it may be provided through glycolysis by the reduction of dihydroxyacetone-phosphate via the NAD^+-coupled glycerol-3-phosphate oxidoreductase present in adipose and in the intestinal mucosa (Fig. 15). In other tissues, including liver, a glycerokinase which catalyzes the reaction between glycerol and ATP is also available as a source of α-glycerophosphate.

Generally, triglyceride synthesis follows the scheme shown in Figure 16. Acylases join two molecules of fatty acyl-CoA to the α' and β positions of α-glycerophosphate in two stages, the first product being lysophosphatidic acid and the second product, phosphatidic acid. In brain, monoglyceride and diglyceride kinases can phosphorylate monoglycerides and diglycerides to lysophosphatidic acid and phosphatidic acid, respectively, with ATP. A

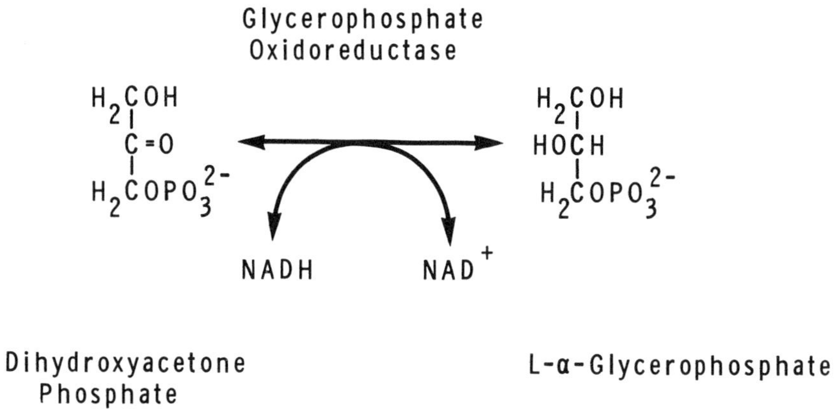

Glycerophosphate
Oxidoreductase

$$
\begin{array}{ccc}
\underset{2}{H_2}\!COH & & \underset{2}{H_2}\!COH \\
C=0 & & HOCH \\
\underset{2}{H_2}\!COPO_3^{2-} & & \underset{2}{H_2}\!COPO_3^{2-}
\end{array}
$$

NADH   NAD$^+$

Dihydroxyacetone   **L-α-Glycerophosphate**
Phosphate

Fig. 15. Conversion of dihydroxyacetone phosphate to α-glycerophosphate. The dihydroxy-acetone phosphate derived from glycolysis thus provides the glycerophosphate for triglyceride biosynthesis.

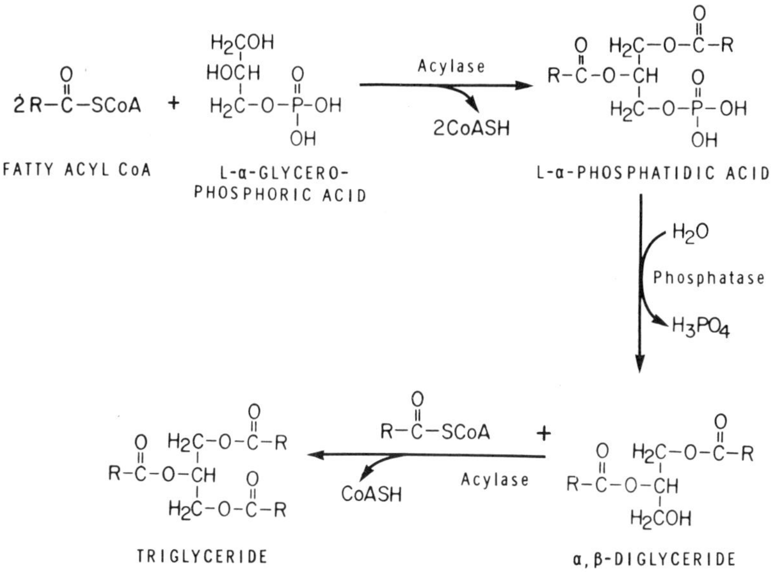

Fig. 16. Triglyceride biosynthesis. This shows the acylation of L-α-glycerophosphoric acid by two molecules of long-chain fatty acyl-CoA (preferably C16 to C18 chain length), followed by a phosphatase-catalyzed cleavage of phosphoric acid from the L-α-phosphatidic acid. The product α,β-diglyceride is acylated once more to the triglyceride. The α and α' positions refer to either of the external carbons of the glycerol moiety, and the β position is the internal, or middle, carbon. Refer to Figure 18 for the various pathways by which phosphatidic acid and the diglyceride are formed.

phosphatase dephosphorylates the phosphatidic acid molecule to the α, β-diglyceride. The diglyceride is acylated further then to the triglyceride. The above reactions are diagrammed in Figure 17.

It has been mentioned previously in connection with lipid digestion, absorption, and transport that pancreatic lipases hydrolyze triglycerides from ingested food to the diglycerides and monoglycerides, as well as to free fatty acids and glycerol, before intestinal absorption occurs. It has also been noted that a large portion of these substrates are reesterified to the triglyceride in the intestinal mucosa. According to the biosynthetic pathway given above, the monoglycerides cannot be acylated directly to the triglyceride, but apparently unique intestinal enzymes exist which catalyze the reactions for production of α, β-diglycerides as shown in Figure 17. The α, β-diglyceride then can be acylated to the triglyceride in the mucosa.

Short- and medium-chain fatty acids are not likely to be esterified to glycerol after intestinal absorption. They enter the portal system to be oxidized by the liver. Esterifying enzymes for long-chain fatty acids in the intestine and liver generally present the pattern of fatty acid distribution to be described, although marked species differences can be detected. The distribution of palmitic acid over the three positions on glycerol appears to be random, but stearic acid prefers an external position. Polyunsaturated fatty acids generally occupy the β, or inner, position as shown in liver and adipose studies. *Cis*-unsaturated fatty acids are esterified more often to the β carbon of glycerol than are the *trans*-unsaturated fatty acids, which appear more often at the α and α′ positions. Experimental evidence points to the fact that hydroxy fatty acids are not substrates for intestinal esterifying enzymes.

Triglyceride Degradation

Triglyceride hydrolysis by lipases occurs for the most part in the small intestine before lipid absorption. Lipases are also responsible for supplying the blood with free fatty acids and glycerol from adipose tissue triglycerides.

Hydrolysis of the α and α′ linkages and of the β linkage of triglycerides appears to be catalyzed by two types of pancreatic lipases which work in the

$$\alpha\text{-Monoglyceride} + \text{Acyl CoA} \xrightarrow{\text{Acylase}} \alpha,\alpha'\text{-Diglyceride} \xleftrightarrow{\text{Isomerase}} \alpha,\beta\text{-Diglyceride}$$

$$\beta\text{-Monoglyceride} + \text{Acyl CoA} \xrightarrow{\text{Acylase}} \alpha,\beta\text{-Diglyceride}$$

Fig. 17. Formation of α,β-diglycerides from α- or β-monoglycerides. These reactions occur uniquely in the intestine and provide for biosynthesis of diglycerides and triglycerides without the involvement of glycerophosphoric acid or of phosphatidic acid.

small intestine. The rapid first steps in triglyceride hydrolysis involve the sequential removal of the α and α' fatty acids. Removal of the β-fatty acid by another type of lipase is slower. The products are simply three fatty acids and one glycerol molecule.

Besides the pancreatic lipases, there are other lipases of adipose, heart muscle, and liver concerned with the transport of lipid into and out of the cell. A lipoprotein lipase, which hydrolyzes only those triglycerides associated with the protein in chylomicrons, appears to be inactive in liver, but active in adipose. The lipoprotein lipases facilitate the transport of fatty acids from triglyceride into the cell where they are immediately reesterified; but whether or not these enzymes necessarily mediate all of triglyceride fatty acid transport into the cell is still an open question. In vivo and in vitro the adipose lipoprotein lipase appears important because increased lipoprotein lipase of rat epididymal fat pads correlates directly with increased lipoprotein triglyceride uptake. Chylomicrons may enter the liver cell intact, conceivably by pinocytosis. The uptake of triglycerides by heart cells also has shown no need of prior hydrolysis.

A hormone-sensitive lipase in adipose and liver tissue, as distinguished from the lipoprotein, lipase, hydrolyzes triglyceride within the cell and is responsible for the blood content of free fatty acids and glycerol. This will be discussed in further detail in the section dealing with hormonal regulation of lipid metabolism.

METABOLISM OF PHOSPHOLIPIDS AND CHOLESTEROL ESTERS

Phospholipids

Only the most important lipids, with respect to their being widely distributed as tissue constituents, will be discussed. These are the lecithins, or phosphatidyl cholines, and the cephalins, or phosphatidyl ethanolamines and phosphatidyl serines. Sphingomyelin is also considered because of its importance in animal metabolism.

The structures of three of the four compounds mentioned above are presented in Figure 2. Phosphatidyl serine resembles phosphatidyl ethanolamine with the exception that a carboxyl group has substituted for one of the hydrogens on the last carbon of the ethanolamine moiety. The phospholipids of the body are continually being built up and broken down, and are probably given their correct functional physiochemical properties through acylation or reacylation with fatty acids of the appropriate length and degree of unsaturation.

The biosynthetic pathways for lecithins and cephalins in animal tissues are presented in Figure 18. The reactions have been shown to be catalyzed by enzymes in the microsomal fraction of various animal organs. The formation of α, β-diglyceride was discussed in connection with triglyceride biosynthesis. The diglyceride usually contains one saturated long-chain (16C or 18C) fatty acid at the α carbon and an unsaturated long-chain fatty acid in the β position. It reacts with cytidine diphosphate-choline (CDP-choline) or CDP-ethanolamine to yield

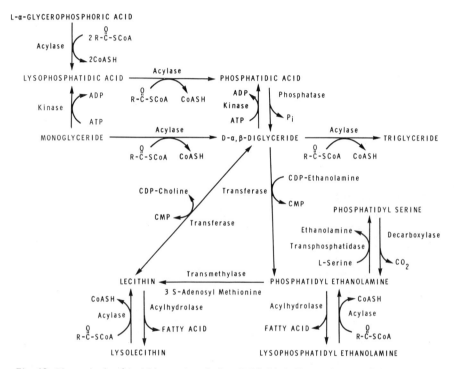

Fig. 18. Biosynthesis of lecithins and cephalins. R-C(=O)- indicates the esterified long-chain fatty acid. L-α-Glycerophosphoric acid is converted to phosphatidic acid after being acylated with two molecules of fatty acyl-CoA. Lysophosphatidic acid is an intermediate in the acylations. A phosphatase cleaves the phosphate moiety from phosphatidic acid to form the α,β-diglyceride, which can be acylated further to the triglyceride. A monoglyceride may be phosphorylated to yield the lysophosphatidic acid; or in a reaction confined to the intestine, a monoglyceride may be acylated directly to the diglyceride. The diglyceride may also react with cytidine diphosphate (CDP) choline to produce phosphatidyl choline (lecithin), or it may be converted to phosphatidyl ethanolamine via CDP-ethanolamine. A transmethylase may convert phosphatidyl ethanolamine to lecithin using three molecules of S-adenosyl methionine. Lecithin may also undergo deacylation to lysolecithin, which in turn can be reacylated with the same or a different fatty acid back to lecithin. Phosphatidyl ethanolamine is capable of undergoing the same types of reactions. By exchanging the ethanolamine group of phosphatidyl ethanolamine for L-serine, a transphosphatidase catalyzes the production of phosphatidyl serine. A decarboxylation of phosphatidyl serine results in regeneration of phosphatidyl ethanolamine. These reactions are associated with the microsomal fraction of the animal cell.

lecithin or phosphatidyl ethanolamine, respectively. Both CDP-esterified compounds are produced by transfer of a cytidyl group from CTP to phosphoryl choline or phosphoryl ethanolamine, previously phosphorylated by ATP. The formation of lecithin in this manner has been demonstrated to be a reversible reaction in liver. S-Adenosyl methionine mediates the methylation of phosphatidyl ethanolamine to lecithin in the liver, while the reaction is negligible in other organs. Alternatively, phosphatidyl ethanolamine may exchange its ethanolamine moiety for L-serine, forming phosphatidyl serine, a compound that after decarboxylation by liver enzymes becomes phosphatidyl ethanolamine. Both lecithin and phosphatidyl ethanolamine can be generated by acylation of the lyso derivatives of these compounds.

The degradation of the phospholipids discussed above is catalyzed by a group of enzymes designated as the phospholipases A, B, C, D and lysophospholipases. In mammalian tissue, the degradation appears to follow a set of reactions, exemplified in lecithin degradation, summarized in Figure 19.

Reaction 1 is catalyzed by phospholipase A_1, which removes the fatty acid at the α position, and reaction 2 shows the action of phospholipase A_2 in removing the β-positioned fatty acid. These phospholipases A are widespread in

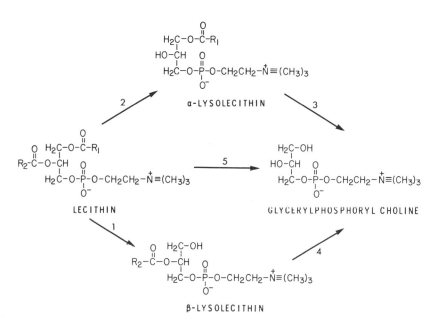

Fig. 19. Degradation of phospholipid in animal tissue. Lecithin is used as an example to illustrate a general set of reactions capable of degrading phospholipids. Reactions 1 and 2 are catalyzed by phospholipases A and A_2 respectively. Reactions 3 and 4 may occur through the action of lysophospholipases, or the reactions possibly may be catalyzed by the phospholipases A. An enzyme designated as phospholipase B may remove both esterified fatty acids as shown in reaction 5.

animal tissues and vary in their relative specificities for substrates as they vary in tissue origin; phospholipase A_2, which resembles snake venom phospholipase, has been detected in rat liver mitochondria, and phospholipase A_1, in rat liver microsomes. In the pancreas, phospholipase A_1 has not been distinguished from pancreatic lipase which splits a fatty acid from the α carbon of triglycerides.

Lysophospholipases, which also are widely distributed through the animal body, may catalyze reactions 3 and 4. Lysophospholipases have been isolated from rat liver microsomes. It is conceivable that the phospholipases A also could catalyze these reactions, and the question as to whether or not they do will have to be resolved by further experimentation.

There have been several reports of an enzyme which removes both the α and β esterified fatty acids of phospholipids, the reaction shown in step 5. These enzymes might be called phospholipase B. Rat liver microsomes and lysosomes, and *Penicillium notatum* have given evidence of containing this type of enzyme.

Phospholipase C has been reported in animal tissue, snake venom, and microorganisms, and phospholipase D has been detected only in plants. Phospholipase D hydrolyzes the phosphodiester linkage between the phosphatidic acid and the nitrogenous base, while phospholipase C hydrolyzes between the α, β-diglyceride and the phosphorylated base. Phosphatidate phosphohydrolase activities have been reported in lysosomes, microsomes, and mitochondria of rat liver.

Sphingomyelins arise from the reactions shown in Figure 20. This synthesis may also proceed via the reaction of CDP-choline with N-acyl-sphingosine.

Sphingosine, shown in Figure 21, and its analog dihydrosphingosine are synthesized in yeast by a condensation of palmityl CoA with L-Serine, dependent on NADPH and pyridoxal phosphate (Braun and Snell).

An enzyme which resembles phospholipase C in activity, but for which lecithin is not a substrate, catalyzes the breakdown of sphingomyelin to N-acylsphingosine and phosphoryl choline. The enzyme has been isolated from rat liver and spleen. In brain, an enzyme exists that will hydrolyze N-acyl-sphingosone to sphingosine and fatty acid.

(1)   Sphingosine + CDP - Choline ⟶ Sphingosylphosphoryl Choline + CMP

(2)   Sphingosylphosphoryl Choline + Acyl CoA ⟶ Sphingomyelin + CoASH

Fig. 20. Biosynthesis of sphingomyelin. The final product may also be generated by the reaction of CDP-choline with N-acyl-sphingosine (ceramide) to yield sphingomyelin and CMP.

Fig. 21. The structural formula of sphingosine. Dihydrosphingosine is the saturated analog of this compound.

Sphingosine

$$CH_3(CH_2)_{12} \quad CH=CH - \underset{\underset{OH}{|}}{CH} - \underset{\underset{NH_2}{|}}{CH} - \underset{\underset{OH}{|}}{CH_2}$$

Cholesterol Esters

The biosynthesis of cholesterol from acetate via the key intermediates mevalonic acid and squalene will not be elaborated upon here; nor will the metabolic scheme for cholesterol degradation or conversion to excretory products. Excellent reviews of these subjects are available in the recent literature (e.g. Bloch).

A transacylase reaction in plasma has been discovered which esterifies cholesterol with the fatty acid removed from the β position of lecithin. Esterification of cholesterol with a fatty acid also occurs in the intestinal mucosa after the free sterol has been absorbed. Dietary cholesterol esters are hydrolyzed in the small intestine before absorption, as are triglycerides.

REGULATION OF LIPID METABOLISM

Control of lipid metabolism depends in great part on the regulation of fatty acid metabolism. The possible points of control are myriad, and it may be that several are in operation simultaneously. For this reason much more intensive research is needed to define clearly the mechanisms by which lipid metabolism fulfills its vital role in the living organism.

Without doubt, the availability or unavailability of glucose as a source of carbon for metabolism has a great deal to do with regulating fatty acid synthesis and oxidation. Closely allied with glucose metabolism are the oxidizing and reducing potentials of the cell. The reducing equivalents supplied by NADPH for fatty acid synthesis and the availability of NAD^+ as an acceptor of reducing equivalents during fatty acid oxidation are absolute necessities. It is logical that an oversupply or sufficiency of reducing power would lead to fatty acid synthesis, and conversely an insufficiency would trigger fatty acid oxidation.

ATP metabolism is associated through oxidative phosphorylation with the production of oxidized and reduced coenzymes for fatty acid oxidation and synthesis. A need for the energy of ATP might well set the lipid metabolism of the cell in the direction of fatty acid oxidation, and an excess of energy could be stored in newly synthesized fatty acids.

Certainly the availability of coenzyme A and cofactors needed for fatty acid activation is required for both synthesis and degradation. Metabolically, fatty acids are relatively inert until they are activated, usually to the fatty acyl-CoA.

Transport across cell membranes must also play an important regulatory role in lipid metabolism. The barrier to acyl-CoA derivatives provided by one of the mitochondrial membranes has been a subject of investigation and will be discussed.

Not least in importance as regulators of lipid metabolism are the activities of the individual enzymes concerned with it. The changes in activity may be brought about by de novo protein synthesis, by inhibition of the enzyme or release of inhibition, or by increased or decreased protein catabolism. All of these possible control centers for lipid metabolism will be discussed in the following paragraphs in light of the influence that diet, metabolic interrelationships, and hormones have on them.

Influence of Diet

Fasting, diabetes, and pancreatectomy, all of which deprive the cell of glucose as a carbon source, result in decreased fatty acid synthesis. Upon further examination, investigators have noticed concomitant activity decreases in key enzymes of lipid metabolism in liver, mammary, and adipose tissue. Some of these enzymes include acetyl-CoA carboxylase, the synthetase complex which converts malonyl-CoA to fatty acids, glucokinase, glucose-6-phosphate dehydrogenase, the citrate cleavage enzyme, malic enzyme, acetate thiokinase, and the desaturase which transforms stearyl-CoA to oleyl-CoA. A high-fat, low-carbohydrate diet decreases acetate incorporation into fatty acids and increases its incorporation into cholesterol. Increased concentration of free fatty acids alone in plasma will cause greater fatty acid oxidation, and the accumulation of palmityl-CoA in the liver inhibits the channeling of acetyl-CoA into fatty acids and into the citric acid cycle, and it stimulates ketogenesis. The small amounts of glucose available in a high-fat diet go to make the α-glycerophosphate for triglyceride synthesis; therefore, it appears that fatty acid synthesis responds readily to glucose availability, while α-glycerophosphate production continues in spite of large alterations in glucose concentration. A high-sodium medium will cause fatty acid synthesis to diminish also.

Enhanced fatty acid synthesis can be induced after starvation by refeeding a high-carbohydrate, low-fat diet. Most of the enzymes mentioned above show an increase over normal activity, which can be prevented by administration of actinomycin or puromycin. This suggests that increased de novo protein synthesis is involved in increased enzyme activity, at least in the later stages of the increase, if not at its initiation. With a high-carbohydrate diet, the rate of α-glycerophosphate synthesis may limit triglyceride formation, since, in adipose tissue, glycerol from lipolysis is not reused for triglyceride synthesis. In a high-potassium medium, an increased bicarbonate concentration will foster increased fatty acid synthesis.

Influence of Metabolic Interrelationships

Ratio of Oxidized to Reduced Coenzymes and ATP Metabolism.   It was discovered that if the conversion of glucose to fatty acids in rat adipose tissue was maximally stimulated by insulin, NADPH production by the pentose cycle and the activity of acetyl-CoA carboxylase were not rate-limiting, but that the limit was probably imposed by the rate of reoxidation of the excess glycolytic NADH, not used for NADPH production by transhydrogenation, via oxidative phosphorylation. The NADH may enter the mitochondrion for oxidative phosphorylation by one of the "shuttle" systems involving either the substrates malate and oxalacetate or the substrates α-glycerophosphate and dihydroxyacetone phosphate.

It can be postulated, therefore, that an overall control of fatty acid synthesis in adipose lies in the rate of high-energy phosphate consumption in the cell, since reoxidation of reduced coenzyme produces ATP as the reducing equivalents proceed down the electron-transport chain to oxygen (Flatt and Ball). For example, the amount of glycolytically produced NADH that is transhydrogenated for synthetic purposes appears to supply a fixed amount, less than 50 percent, of the NADPH for fatty acid synthesis. The pentose phosphate cycle, fluctuating concomitantly with the rate of lipogenesis, probably supplies the balance of the NADPH. If the cell rapidly consumes its high-energy phosphate, then the oxidative phosphorylation process may rapidly reoxidize glycolytic NADH not used for transhydrogenation, since excess ATP is removed. Reoxidation of NADH, in turn, allows a greater conversion of glycolytic triosephosphates to acetyl-CoA, thus providing more substrate for an increased fatty acid synthesis.

As was mentioned in connection with mitochondrial fatty acid synthesis, perhaps all mitochondria possess a fatty acid synthesis-oxidation cycle regulated by the intramitochondrial ratio of NADH to NAD^+. Reducing equivalents from NADH not in demand for ATP synthesis can be available for fatty acid synthesis. Succinate is a singularly potent stimulator of fatty acid synthesis in rabbit sarcosomes, and it also generates immediately a large supply of NADH via reversed electron flow from succinyl-CoA to FAD^+ to NAD^+. The resulting high NADH : NAD^+ ratio then is able to direct the cycle toward synthesis (Whereat et al.). Excess amounts of intermediates of the citric acid cycle can inhibit fatty acid oxidation by competing for NAD^+, and conversely it appears that a large supply of fatty acids for oxidation will cause an increase in the concentration of the reduced partner of NAD^+-coupled substrate pairs.

Fatty Acid Activation. In connection with the role of fatty acid activation as a regulator of lipid metabolism, it should be noted that fatty acid activation may occur by one of two or more postulated routes that have been studied in rat liver and brain mitochondria and in rat liver microsomes. The first pathway is dependent on coenzyme A and ATP for forming fatty acyl-CoA; the second one appears to require a fatty acyl high-energy intermediate, generated by the electron-transport chain, for fatty acyl-CoA formation; and a possible third mechanism of fatty acid oxidation exists which involves no fatty acyl-CoA. Rat liver mitochondria will oxidize acyl-carnitine in preference to pyruvate. Since both reactions require coenzyme A, the suppression of pyruvate oxidation may indicate competition for coenzyme A in mitochondria.

Transport Across Mitochondrial Membranes. Carnitine derivatives of fatty acids or of acetate seem to be one answer to the problem of their transport across the mitochondrial membrane, along with the citrate cleavage enzyme. The relationship between citrate cleavage enzyme and acetate transport has been considered along with carbon sources for fatty acid synthesis. The relationship of carnitine to fatty acid synthesis has been mentioned also when sources of carbon for synthesis were considered. Further support for the transport of acetyl-carnitine out of the mitochondrion for cytoplasmic fatty acid synthesis from acetyl-CoA comes from the finding that carnitine stimulates the conversion of glucose, but not of citrate, to fatty acids in isolated liver and in vivo. With respect to the relationship between carnitine and fatty acid oxidation, it is certain that cytoplasmic fatty acids must enter the mitochondrion for oxidation, and they may do so via a reaction similar to that given in Figure 8, with fatty acyl-carnitine being produced on the external side of the mitochondrial membrane and fatty acyl-CoA being regenerated intramitochondrially. This transfer has been called the rate-limiting step of fatty acid oxidation. Carnitine itself stimulates fatty acid oxidation.

Ninety percent of the carnitine-palmityl transferase is located in the mitochondrial cell fraction, and its activity increases under conditions that increase fatty acid oxidation and correlates well with the ability of the tissue to oxidize fatty acids. Carnitine-acetyl transferase has been found in both the mitochondrial and supernatant cell fractions. Studies of mitochondrial structure as it is involved in lipid metabolism reveal that the outer, more permeable membrane contains the enzymes for fatty acid activation—e.g., fatty acid thiokinase—and the inner membrane vectorially carries the carnitine-acyl transferase which transports fatty acids into the mitochondrial matrix for oxidation. It even can be inferred from some experimental results that there exist an outer pool of carnitine-acyl transferases accessible to acyl-CoA and an inner pool for acyl carnitine derivatives (Tubbs and Garland).

Palmityl-carnitine enhances the rate of fatty acid synthesis in rat liver supernatant, presumably by reversing the feedback inhibition effected by long-chain acyl-CoA. As would be expected, carnitine affects several other aspects of lipid and carbohydrate metabolism, probably through its property of accepting acyl units from coenzyme A.

Enzyme Stimulation and Inhibition.   Regulation of enzyme activity is another means of controlling lipid metabolism. For example, it was found that phosphate sugars, especially fructose-1,6-diphosphate, stimulate fatty acid synthesis. The possible mechanisms of the action include an allosteric stimulation of the transacylases, the condensing enzyme, or the dehydrase, or the phosphate sugars might assist the synthetase complex in maintaining an active configuration. The phosphate group on the sugars must be important, since a high inorganic phosphate concentration by itself will cause the stimulation (Wakil et al.).

The stimulation and feedback inhibition of acetyl-CoA carboxylase by polycarboxylic acids and fatty acyl-CoA, respectively, has been discussed with carbon sources for fatty acid synthesis. The aggregation or disassociation of the enzyme's three protein subunits may be the mechanism through which the stimulatory and inhibitory effects work. The stimulation of fatty acid synthesis in rat liver and mammary gland preparations by added microsomes may operate through binding the fatty acids, thus relieving feedback inhibition on acetyl-CoA carboxylase. To substantiate this theory, it was discovered that microsomal stimulation could be imitated by purified acetyl-CoA carboxylase and that the microsomal stimulation occurs only when acetyl-CoA or acetate is used as substrate for fatty acid synthesis (Lorch et al.). However, a liver slice preparation from a fasted animal demonstrated a large decrease in fatty acid synthetase activity, accompanied by only half as large a decrease in acetyl-CoA carboxylase activity, leaving the conclusion to be drawn that, in the intact cell, decreased carboxylase activity cannot account entirely for the lowered fatty acid synthesis.

The free fatty acid inhibition of glucose-6-phosphate dehydrogenase was extrapolated to physiologic concentrations, and the conclusion drawn that only long term contact with fatty acids in vivo inhibits the enzyme which is involved in cytoplasmic NADPH production. The fatty acids do not appear to be immediate inhibitors of glucose-6-phosphate dehydrogenase in vivo (Shafrir et al.). Recent experiments have demonstrated that long-chain fatty acids, such as palmitic acid, are noncompetitive inhibitors of purified bovine adrenal glucose-6 -phosphate dehydrogenase (Criss and McKerns) and that palmityl CoA inhibits the same enzyme in rat liver and yeast (Taketa and Pogell).

Influence of Hormones

The effects exerted by hormones on lipid metabolism will be examined from the point of view of enhancement or inhibition of the various main processes of lipid metabolism such as fatty acid synthesis, oxidation, modification (e.g., desaturation), triglyceride synthesis, and lipolysis.

Fatty Acid Synthesis. Insulin is certainly the hormone most involved with fat deposition in general; insulin stimulates the flow of glucose through all the pathways open to it, including glycogen synthesis, glycolysis, the pentose cycle, fatty acid synthesis, and glycerol formation. It also directly enhances the entry of glucose into the cell. Whether or not insulin has any direct effect on the enzymes of fatty acid synthesis remains unknown. Insulin stimulation of fatty acid synthesis occurs only in the presence of glucose or a derivative of it.

A prolactin preparation, possibly contaminated with growth hormone, was found to enhance fatty acid synthesis promptly in pigeon liver both in vivo and in vitro (Goodridge and Ball). The enhancement depends on adequate carbohydrate intake. Estrogen stimulates the incorporation of the label of glucose-1-H^3 into lipids of adipose tissue isolated from female rats. Estrogens also have a synergistic effect with insulin in stimulating lipid synthesis from glucose in adipose tissue (Gilmour and McKerns). Thyroxin also appears to be necessary to maintain a normal level of lipogenesis.

As would be expected, diabetes and pancreatectomy both will result in decreased fatty acid and sterol synthesis in the liver and this decrease is thought to be a result of lowered enzyme level rather than a limitation imposed by NADPH supply or an enzyme inhibition (Dahlen et al.). Hypophysectomized rats also demonstrate a decreased fatty acid synthesis in the liver along with diminished citrate cleavage enzyme activity. These decreases cannot be repaired by refeeding a high-carbohydrate diet. In addition, thyroidectomized animals show decreased lipogenesis, possibly caused by an inhibitory change in the redox state of the nicotinamide adenine nucleotides and by a total decrease in their amounts (Walters and McLean).

Fatty Acid Oxidation. Long-chain fatty acid oxidation, as measured by the conversion of palmitate-1-C^{14} to $C^{14}O_2$, was stimulated by ovine growth hormone in isolated fat pads of hypophysectomized rats. Even carnitine-acyl transferase activity, a probable rate-limiting step of fatty acid oxidation, showed an increase under these conditions.

Desaturation. Both insulin and thyroxin have been found to stimulate desaturase activity; in fact, the desaturases that convert stearic acid to oleic acid and linoleic acid to γ-linolenic acid in rats depend on insulin for their induction at the mRNA level. Thyroxin also increases the amount of oleic acid in liver and is able to repair the lost desaturase activity in diabetic animals. In vitro, thyroxin causes a stimulation of desaturase activity in liver slices and microsomes. Diethyl stilbestrol, a synthetic estrogen analog, will decrease desaturase activity in adipose tissue.

Lipolysis. Adipose tissue appears to be the large target for some of the fatty acid mobilizing hormones that stimulate lipolysis. The resultant release of free fatty acids from within the adipose cell by hormone-sensitive lipase causes increased fatty acid oxidation and changes in glucose metabolism of the body.

The lipolytic hormones, which effect a rapid but nonpersistent response, appear to act through cyclic 3′,5′-AMP which activates the adipose lipase. The effect of these hormones has been pinpointed to a stimulation of adenyl cyclase, which forms cyclic AMP from ATP, rather than to an inhibition of the phosphodiesterase which transforms cyclic AMP to 5'-AMP. These lipolytic hormones include, among others, the catecholamines, epinephrine and norepinephrine, whose primary target is adipose tissue. In addition, luteinizing hormone, ACTH, thyroid-stimulating hormone, and glucagon stimulate lipolysis in rat adipose tissue in vitro. However, the effect requires a high and possibly unphysiologic concentration of the hormones. Glucocorticoids stimulate an increase in the release of free fatty acids from adipose tissue. The increased level of free fatty acids decreases the utilization of glucose in the liver. Cortisol and other glucocorticoids potentiate the epinephrine effect probably through an inhibition of free fatty acid esterification rather than a stimulation of lipolysis.

The lipolytic hormone eliciting a slow, sustained response in adipose tissue is growth hormone. Only after several hours of in vitro incubation can the growth hormone effect be demonstrated. The effect can be prevented by actinomycin, an inhibitor of protein synthesis, and puromycin, an inhibitor of RNA synthesis. Since an intact pituitary is also required for the rapid-acting lipolytic hormones to exert their action, several investigators have reasoned that growth hormone stimulates additional lipase (protein) synthesis.

Insulin causes a decrease in cyclic AMP in vitro in adipose tissue, and perhaps it is through this mechanism that insulin inhibits adipose lipolytic activity in vitro and in vivo in pancreatectomized rats. A direct correlation has been shown between insulin's antilipolytic activity and its action on lowering the level of cyclic 3',5'-AMP. However, normal rats in vivo respond to insulin with increased lipolysis, caused possibly by insulin stimulation of a lipase-activating pancreatic factor. Insulin's antilipolytic activity on adipose tissue of alloxan-diabetic and of fasting rats may be a direct cause of the prompt suppression of hepatic gluconeogenesis. In other words, when the supply of free fatty acids, which stimulate gluconeogenesis, becomes small through decreased lipolysis, gluconeogenesis diminishes.

Prostaglandin $E_1(PGE_1)$ decreases the lipolytic action of ephinephrine, thyroid stimulating hormone, ACTH and glucagon on adipose tissue. It is possible that PGE_1 inhibits the adenyl cyclase system. Polyunsaturated fatty acids such as arachidonic can serve as precursors for prostaglandin synthesis in many tissues. Their biosynthesis, structures, and properties have been reviewed (Bergstrom and Samuelson).

Growth hormone will increase fatty acid incorporation into triglycerides and into phospholipids in the isolated epididymal fat pad of hypophysectomized rats.

A Homeostatic Situation

To summarize the regulation of lipid metabolism, an example of homeostasis in a normal individual when a drop in blood glucose occurs as a result of starvation or reduced carbohydrate intake will be considered. As explained in Chapter 3 (see Figure 1), lowered blood sugar signals the release of epinephrine from the adrenal medulla. Two of the several effects of epinephrine are stimulation of ACTH secretion by the pituitary and an indirect activation of lipases in adipose tissue. ACTH stimulates the adrenal cortex to secrete glucocorticoids which inhibit protein synthesis in tissues other than liver, thus increasing the amino acid pool available to the liver. Since the supply of glucose is limited, certain of the amino acids then may become the principal source of pyruvate through transamination reactions. The lipases in adipose cause breakdown of the triglycerides stored there, and the resulting free fatty acids tend to have a glucose sparing effect by inhibiting glycolytic enzymes. These same fatty acids are oxidized in several tissues of the body, but here will be considered to be transported to the liver, where a large portion of β-oxidation occurs.

During mitochondrial oxidation in the liver, the fatty acids may supply adequate acetyl-CoA for ATP generation through the citric acid cycle if additional ATP is needed over that derived from reoxidation of the coenzymes reduced during fatty acid oxidation. Fatty acid oxidation may also increase the pool of acetyl-CoA to the point where pyruvate (now being generated from the amino acid pool) needs no longer to contribute to it. Thus, pyruvate may be shunted into oxalacetate production (and gluconeogenesis). This could occur in several ways. The excess acetyl-CoA derived from fatty acid oxidation could inhibit the conversion of pyruvate to acetyl-CoA. Fatty acid oxidation would increase the supply of the acetyl-CoA for the pyruvate carboxylase reaction yielding oxalacetate. Increased acetyl-CoA could increase citrate production via the citrate condensing enzyme. Citrate inhibits phosphofructokinase, which is a controlling enzyme for glycolysis. Oxalacetate, possibly previously limited by a partial shutdown of the citric acid cycle due to efficient ATP generation by fatty acid oxidation, then becomes available for gluconeogenic reactions operating through phosphoenolpyruvate to glucose. There is also evidence that glucocorticoids may induce the gluconeogenic enzymes.

Beyond these reactions, the acetyl-CoA pool may still contain an oversupply, in which case excess molecules of acetyl-CoA condense in pairs to yield excess acetoacetate, the basis for ketosis.

Thus a summary view of this homeostatic mechanism reveals that under conditions where glucose for metabolism is limited, the cell does all it can to spare the glucose present and to enhance its supply. The free fatty acids released by lipolysis shut off glycolysis to some extent, thereby preserving the available glucose. Pyruvate, usually an intermediate of glycolysis, is now derived from an increased amino acid pool in the liver. The acetyl-CoA pool becomes larger through increased fatty acid oxidation and allows its precursor, pyruvate, to be shunted to oxalacetate production. Since the citric acid cycle, of which oxalacetate is an intermediate, may be partially shut down owing to efficient ATP generation through fatty acid oxidation, the oxalacetate from pyruvate, not needed for the cycle, may be used for gluconeogenic reactions. Oxalacetate can be reduced in liver mitochondria to malate. Malate diffuses out, and in the cytoplasm is converted to oxalacetate along with the reduction of NAD^+. Thus, malate acts as a carrier of reducing equivalents between mitochondria and cytoplasm. NADH supplies hydrogen for the conversion of 1,3-diphosphoglycerate to glyceraldehyde-3-phosphate during gluconeogenesis (see Fig. 10, Chapter 3). Oxalacetate is transformed to phosphoenolpyruvate and eventually yields glucose.

ANSELL, G.B., and HAWTHORNE, J.N. *Phospholipids.* Amsterdam, Elsevier, 1964.
BERGSTROM, S., and SAMUELSON, B. *Prostaglandins.* Stockholm, Interscience Publishers, 1967.
CLAYTON, R.B. Biosynthesis of sterols, steroids, and terpenoids. *Quart Rev,* 19:168, 1965.
DANIELSSON, H., and TCHEN, T.T. Steroid metabolism. *In* Greenberg, D.M., ed. *Metabolic Pathways,* 3rd ed. New York, Academic Press, 1968, Vol. 2, pp. 117-168.
FRANTZ, I.D., Jr., and SCHROEPFER, G.J., Jr. Sterol biosyntheses. *Ann Rev Biochem,* 36:691, 1967.
GREEN, D.E., and ALLMAN, D.W. Biosynthesis of fatty acids. *In* Greenberg, D.M., ed. *Metabolic Pathways,* 3rd ed. New York, Academic Press, 1968, Vol. 2, pp. 37-67.
——Fatty Acid Oxidation. *In* Greenberg, D.M., ed. *Metabolic Pathways,* 3rd ed. New York, Academic Press, 1968, Vol. 2, pp. 1-36.
GOODMAN, DeW. S. Cholesterol ester metabolism. *Physiol Rev,* 45:747, 1965.
KENNEDY, E.P. Biosynthesis of complex lipids. *Fed Proc,* 20:934, 1961.
MAHLER, H.R., and CORDES, E.H. *Biological Chemistry.* New York, Harper & Row, 1966.
MASORO, E.J. Mechanisms related to the homeostatic regulation of lipogenesis. *Ann NY Acad Sci,* 131:199, 1965.
OLSON, J.A. Lipid metabolism. *Ann Rev Biochem,* 35:559, 1966.
ROSSITER, R.J. Metabolism of phosphatides. *In* Greenberg, D.M., ed. *Metabolic Pathways,* 3rd ed. New York, Academic Press, 1968, Vol. 2, pp. 69-115.
SHAFRIR, E. Adipose tissue and neonatal homeostasis. *Israel J Med Sci,* 4:277, 1968.
SHAPIRO, B. Lipid metabolism. *Ann Rev Biochem,* 36:247, 1967.
VAGELOS, P.R. Lipid metabolism. *Ann Rev Biochem,* 33:139, 1964.
van DEENEN, L.L.M., and de HASS, G.H. Phosphoglycerides and phospholipases. *Ann Rev Biochem,* 35:157, 1966.
WHITE, A., HANDLER, P., and SMITH, E.L. *Principles of Biochemistry.* New York, McGraw-Hill Book Co., Inc., 1964.

Specific References

BALL, E.G. Regulation of fatty acid synthesis in adipose tissue. *Advances Enzyme Regulat,* 4:3, 1966.

BLOCH, K. The biological synthesis of cholesterol. *Science*, 150:19, 1965.

BRAUN, P.E., and SNELL, E.E. Biosynthesis of sphingolipid bases. II. Keto intermediates in synthesis of sphingosine and dihydrosphingosine by cell-free extracts of *Hansensula ciferri*. *J Biol Chem*, 143:3775, 1968.

CANTAROW, A., and SCHEPARTZ, B. *Biochemistry*, 3rd ed. Philadelphia, W.B. Saunders Co., 1962, p. 33.

CHANG, H.C., SEIDMAN, I., TEEBOR, G., and LANE, M.D. Liver acetyl CoA carboxylase and fatty acid synthetase: relative activities in the normal state and in hereditary obesity. *Biochem Biophys Res Commun*, 28:682, 1967.

CHRIST, E.J.V.J. Fatty acid synthesis in mitochondria. Elongation of short-chain fatty acids and formation of unsaturated long-chain fatty acids. *Biochim Biophys Acta*, 152:50, 1968.

CRISS, W.E., and McKERNS, K.W. Unpublished observations.

DAHLEN, J.V., KENNAN, A.L., and PORTER, J.W. Effect of alloxan and portacaval shunt on the synthesis of fatty acids and sterols by rat liver. *Arch Biochem*, 124:51, 1968.

DAS, M.L., ORRENIUS, S., and ERNSTER, L. On the fatty acid and hydrocarbon hydroxylation in rat liver microsomes. *Europ J Biochem*, 4:519, 1968.

FLATT, J.P., and BALL, E.G. Studies on the metabolism of adipose tissue. XIX. An evaluation of the major pathways of glucose catabolism as influenced by acetate in the presence of insulin. *J Biol Chem*, 241:2862, 1966.

FOSTER, D.W., and SRERE, P.A. Citrate cleavage enzyme and fatty acid synthesis. *J Biol Chem*, 243:1926, 1968.

GILMAUR, K.E., and McKERNS, K.W. Insulin and estrogen regulation of lipid synthesis in adipose tissue. *Biochim Biophys Acta*, 116:220, 1966.

GOODRIDGE, A.G. Induction of lipogenesis, malic enzyme and citrate cleavage enzyme in liver of newly-hatched chicks. *Fed Proc*, 27, Abstract 3388, 1968.

HARLAN, W.R., Jr., and WAKIL, S.J. The pathways of synthesis of fatty acids by mitochondria. *Biochem Biophys Res Commun*, 8:131, 1962.

KREBS, H.A. The regulation of the release of ketone bodies by the liver. *Advances Enzym Regulat*, 4:339, 1966.

LORCH, E., ABRAHAM, S., and CHAIKOFF, I.L. Fatty acid synthesis in complex systems. The possibility of regulation by microsomes. *Biochim Biophys Acta*, 70:627, 1963.

LYNEN, F. The role of biotin-dependent carboxylations in biosynthetic reactions. *Biochem J*, 102:381, 1967.

MATTHES, K.J., ABRAHAM, S., and CHAIKOFF, I.L. Hydrogen transfer in fatty acid synthesis by rat liver and mammary gland cell-free preparations studied with tritium-labeled pyridine nucleotides and glucose. *Biochim Biophys Acta*, 70:242, 1963.

SHAFRIR, E., LAURIS, V., and CAHILL, G.F., Jr. Free fatty acid (FFA) inhibition of glucose-6-phosphate dehydrogenase (G6PDH) in liver and adipose tissue. Fed Proc, 27, Abstract 653, 1968.

TAKETA, K., and POGELL, B.M. The effect of palmityl coenzyme A on glucose-6-phosphate dehydrogenase and other enzymes. *J Biol Chem*, 241:720, 1966.

TUBBS, P.K., and GARLAND, P.B. Membranes and fatty acid metabolism. *Brit Med Bull*, 24:158, 1968.

WAKIL, S.J., GOLDMAN, J.K., WILLIAMSON, I.P., and TOOMEY, R.E. Stimulation of fatty acid biosynthesis by phosphorylated sugars. *Proc Nat Acad Sci USA*, 55:880, 1966.

WALTERS, E., and McLEAN, P. Effect of thyroidectomy on pathways of glucose metabolism in lactating rat mammary gland. *Biochem J*, 105:615, 1967.

WHEREAT, A.F., HULL, F.E., and ORISHIMO, M.W. The role of succinate in the regulation of fatty acid synthesis by heart mitochondria. *J Biol Chem*, 242:4013, 1967.

10

Genetic Control of Metabolism

The function of a tissue cell is determined basically by the genetic material in the sense that the genetic material regulates not only the synthesis of structural protein, but also the enzyme proteins that determine metabolic function. A cell will have a spectrum of enzymes, genetically determined, limiting its ability to metabolize substrates or synthesize products. However, in the case of some organs, function may not be completely realized in the absence of certain hormones. Thus, hormones may modify the genetic expression of cell function and replication. There are a number of possible ways hormones may do this. They may modify the activity of enzymes involved in metabolism of the cell or in the synthesis of DNA or RNA; or in other ways they may regulate the synthesis of RNA or of proteins synthesized against messenger RNA (mRNA).

The main genetic material of higher organisms is nucleic acid in the form of a double helical deoxyribonucleic acid (DNA), which can be replicated during cell division. In addition, each "unit of function", or gene, of the DNA molecule serves as a template for the synthesis of a complementary copy of the gene in the form of mRNA. The mRNA in turn is a sequence of three nucleotides (codon), each codon specifing an amino acid. The amino acid sequence of the polypeptide chain of the protein is assembled in a special way controlled by the purine and pyrimidine base sequences of the mRNA, as will be shown later in this chapter. DNA is found chiefly in the nucleus and appears to be localized in the chromosomes. DNA has also been found in mitochondria. RNA is associated with organelles of the cell as well as existing free in the cytoplasm. DNA increases during cell division, but otherwise is constant in the somatic cells irrespective of the function or metabolic activity of the cell. RNA, on the other hand, increases as metabolic activity increases. A simple concept of the control of polypeptide synthesis is outlined in Figure 1. These concepts will be

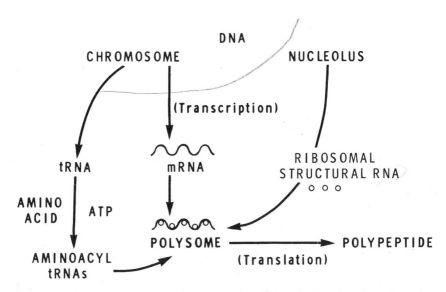

Fig. 1. Chromosomes are made up of a great number of genes in the cell nucleus. A gene is a sequence of genetic material consisting of numerous purine and pyrimidine nucleotides which eventually is expressed as a single polypeptide. The genes serve as templates for the synthesis of various types of RNA such as messenger RNA or transfer RNA. For a messenger RNA (mRNA), a gene serves as a template for the synthesis (transcription) of a complementary structure of triplets of nucleotides (codons) which can bind specific transfer RNA's (tRNA's). Each tRNA carries a specific amino acid as an aminoacyl-tRNA. The amino acids are incorporated into polypeptide chains in a sequence (translation) according to the sequence of codons in the mRNA.

Ribosomal structural RNA is synthesized in the nucleolus and, along with protein, forms the ribonucleoprotein particles, and ribosomes in the cytoplasm. The ribosomes attach to each strand of mRNA, forming a polyribosome, where protein synthesis takes place. Each polysome synthesizes a polypeptide chain as the mRNA moves over the ribosomes. Growth of the polypeptide chain occurs sequentially from the amino end to the final carboxyl end. Each of 20 possible amino acids is carried to the site of polypeptide synthesis by a specific tRNA having a recognition site for an activating enzyme specific for a particular amino acid.

The tRNA as an aminoacyl-tRNA, also has a coding site of three nucleotides which is complementary to the codon on the mRNA which represents the amino acid.

Thus, the base sequence of DNA is transcribed to a complementary mRNA containing codons that determine the amino acid sequence of the polypeptide. These concepts will be developed in a stepwise fashion in the text.

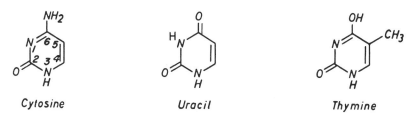

Cytosine   Uracil   Thymine

Fig. 2. Pyrimidine bases. The numbering system shown is one analogous to the pyrimidine portion of purine shown in Figure 3. In the newer Chemical Abstracts System numbering starts with the bottom ring nitrogen and proceeds clockwise. The predominent tautomer form of the pyrimidine and purine bases is shown in Figures 2 and 3, except for thymine. The usual form of thymine is equivalent to the one shown for uracil. Normal base pairing of the predominent tautomer forms is shown in Figures 8 and 9. Rarer tautomers are a potential cause of mutations or aging.

developed as the chapter proceeds. First we should consider briefly the components and synthesis of polynucleic acids such as DNA and RNA.

NUCLEOSIDES AND NUCLEOTIDES

DNA and RNA consist of numerous nucleosides linked together by phosphoric acid. Nucleosides are made up of purine or pyrimidine bases linked through a C-N bond to ribose in the case of RNA, or deoxyribose sugars in the case of DNA. The main pyrimidine bases are cytosine, uracil, and thymine (Fig. 2). RNA contains mainly cytosine and uracil; DNA of higher animals contains cytosine and thymine. The two principal purine bases in RNA and DNA are adenine and guanine, the structures of which are shown in Figure 3.

The pentose sugars of the nucleosides are riboses in the form of a furanose ring with the hydroxyls on carbon-1' *trans* (β) to the hydroxyl on carbon-2' or -3'. The structures of ribose and deoxyribose are shown in Figure 4.

In a pyrimidine nucleoside, such as uridine, the base and sugar are linked by an N-glycoside bond between carbon-1' of the sugar and the nitrogen at

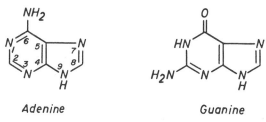

Adenine   Guanine

Fig. 3. Purine bases.

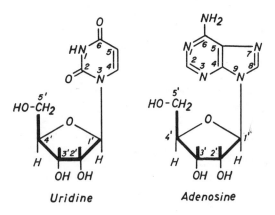

β-D-Ribose β-D-Deoxyribose

Fig. 4. Ribose and deoxyribose sugars.

position 3 of the pyrimidine. In a purine nucleoside, such as adenosine, the C-N bond is between carbon-1' of the sugar and the nitrogen in position 9 of the purine. These structures are illustrated in Figure 5.

Nucleosides have names derived from their bases; pyrimidine derivatives end in -idine and purines in -osine

Base	Nucleoside
Cytosine	Cytidine
Uracil	Uridine
Thymine	Thymidine
Adenine	Adenosine
Guanine	Guanosine

Nucleotides are the phosphoric acid esters of the nucleosides. Esters at the 5' position of the ribose or deoxyribose moiety are the important biological nucleotides. Other phosphoric acid esters of the free hydroxyl groups of the sugars are possible.

Uridine   Adenosine

Fig. 5. Nucleosides.

The biosynthesis of the parent pyrimidine nucleotide uridine-5'-phosphate begins with the formation of orotic acid from carbamyl phosphate and aspartic acid. Orotic acid reacts with 5-phosphoribosyl pyrophosphate under the direction of the enzyme orotidine-5'-pyrophosphorylase to give orotidine-5'-phosphate, which is enzymatically decarboxylated to give uridine-5'-phosphate, as shown in Figure 6.

Free uracil and ribose-1-phosphate can also be enzymatically converted to the nucleoside uridine and, when phosphorylated at the 5' position of the sugar moiety, can form uridine-5'-phosphate. The phosphorylated ribose sugars, such as phosphoribosyl pyrophosphate and ribose-1-phosphate, are derived from ribose-5-phosphate. The principal source of ribose-5-phosphate is probably the metabolism of glucose-6-phosphate by the pentose phosphate cycle.

Uridine-5'-phosphate with adenosinetriphosphate (ATP) and a kinase can form 5'-diphosphates and 5'-triphosphates. The other pyrimidine derivatives arise from these phosphorylated uridine derivatives. For example, uridine-5'-triphosphate becomes cytidine triphosphate with the enzymatic conversion of the C-6 hydroxyl of the pyrimidine ring to an amino group. In addition, deoxyribose derivatives can form from the 5'-diphosphate ribose compounds by loss of the oxygen at the 2' position of the ribose.

The biosynthesis of the parent purine nucleotide, inosinic acid, occurs in a different fashion from the synthesis of pyrimidine nucleotides. The formation of the purine ring system takes place on the sugar-phosphate component, 5-phosphoribosylamine, which is derived from 5-phosphoribosyl pyrophosphate and glutamine. Adenosine-5'-phosphate (adenylic acid) and guanosine-5' phosphate (guanylic acid) are derived from inosinic acid.

DNA consists of a very large polynucleotide molecule of equal proportions of purine and pyrimidine bases such that adenine plus guanine equals thymine plus cytosine. The sugar residues of the nucleotides are linked by their phosphate moieties in such a way that the C-3' position of one deoxyribose is linked to the C-5' position of the next. A trinucleotide fragment is shown in Figure 7.

Wilkins and Randle and Franklin and Gosling revealed by x-ray diffraction analysis of various DNA molecules that the flat structures of the pyrimidine and purine bases are arranged at right angles to the long axis of the polynucleotide chain, each base being separated from its neighbor by 3.44 Å. The long axis of the chain forms a sugar-phosphate "backbone." They also showed that the chain is wound helically around a central axis with one full turn of the helix extending 34 Å. In addition, according to Watson and Crick (see also Crick and Watson), DNA is a double helix of two long strands of polynucleotide. The two strands are held together by hydrogen bonds between base pairs facing in toward one another in such a way that the purine base, adenine, forms a hydrogen bond with the complement pyrimidine, thymine, while guanine pairs with cytosine. A hydrogen bond is essentially a proton shared between two electron pairs from

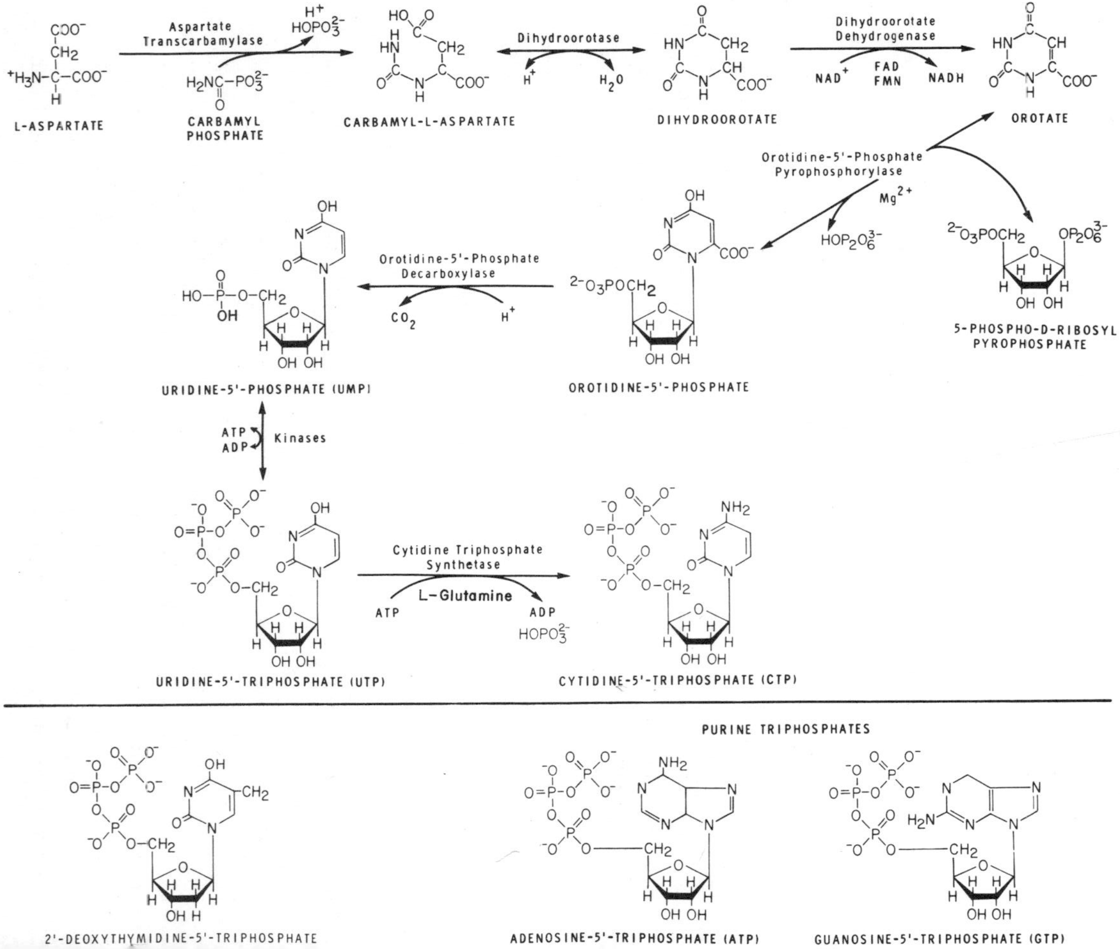

Fig. 6. The formation of the parent, pyrimidine nucleotide, uridine-5'-phosphate from orotate and 5-phosphoribosyl pyrophosphate. The triphosphate (UTP) can be formed from this. Cytidine-5'-triphosphate is formed from UTP. UTP and CTP are the two principal pyrimidine compounds used in the synthesis of RNA in higher animals, while DNA utilizes 2'-deoxycytidine-5'-triphosphate and 2'-deoxythymidine-5'-triphosphate. The thymine base for this latter compound is illustrated. Also indicated are the two principal purine triphosphates of RNA. Again, DNA uses 2-deoxy derivatives.

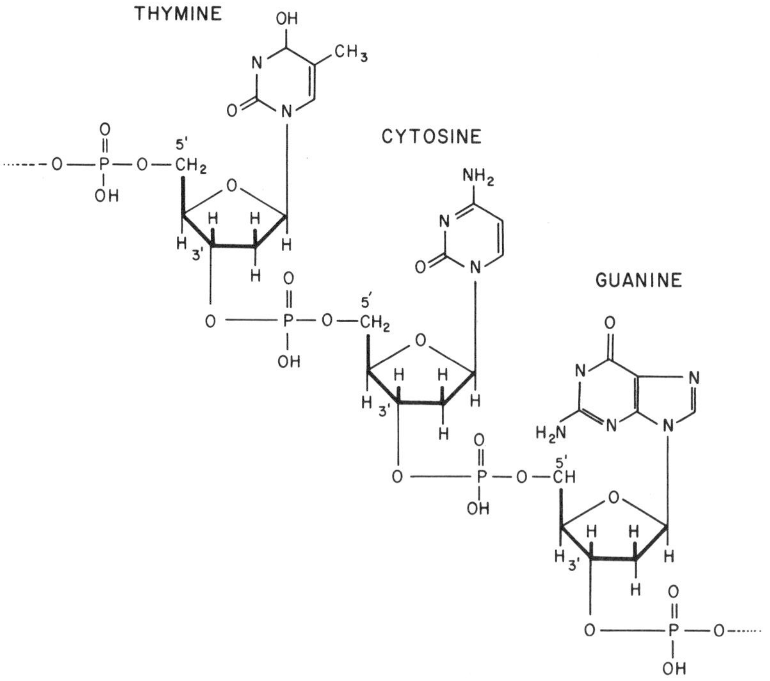

Fig. 7. The phosphate linkage between the 3' and 5' positions of the deoxyribose sugars in a polynucleotide.

different atoms. The base pairing of adenine and thymine is shown in Figure 8, and the H-bond pairing of cytosine and guanine in Figure 9.

REPLICATION OF DNA

The DNA molecule consists of two polynucleotide chains wound around each other to form a double helix. The specific forces holding the two chains together are principally the hydrogen bonds between adenine and thymine and between cytosine and guanine. In addition, van der Waals forces between the hydrophobic bases contribute to the maintenance of a rigid structure.

The pairing of the bases is an essential part of the process of replication, allowing each chain, as it unwinds, to act as a template for the synthesis of a complementary chain of bases that coils around each original chain. There is evidence that unwinding of the original helix proceeds down the chain, followed closely by the synthesis and coiling of the new strand with the old. Thus, when the original DNA is completely unwound, a replica is formed. Each double helix

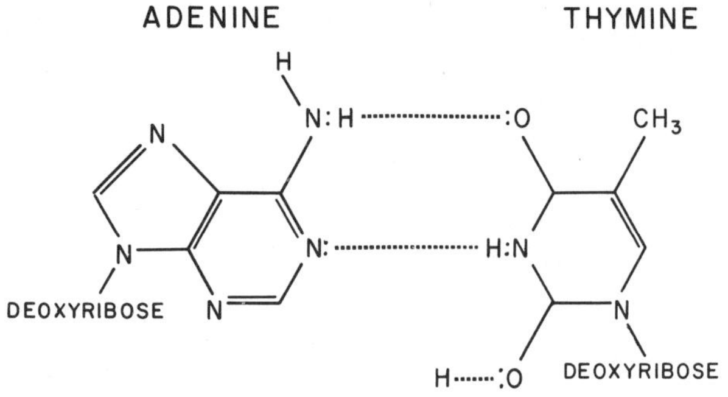

Fig. 8. Hydrogen bonding between the base pairs adenine (A) and thymine (T). These two bases form the complementary pair A-T. The proton (H) from the amine group of adenine can be shared with an electron lone pair on the oxygen atom in thymine. The proton on N at position 1 in thymine is shared with the electron lone pair on N_1 of adenine. In RNA, uracil takes the place of thymine.

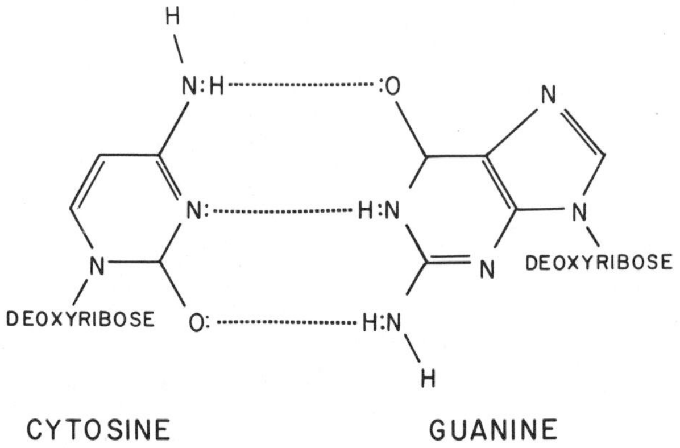

Fig. 9. Hydrogen bonding between the base pairs cytosine (C) and guanine (G). Three protons are shared between three electron lone pairs on atoms as shown, to form the complementary base pair G-C.

then consists of an original and a new complementary strand. This theory for the replication of DNA is called the "Y mechanism" and is illustrated in Figure 10. It is not clear how the orderly unwinding, replication, and rewinding of the parent and daughter chains are achieved and controlled, or how the energy is supplied (Crick).

The replication of a DNA molecule in vitro was first achieved by Kornberg. An enzyme, DNA polymerase, isolated from *Escherichia coli* was found to replicate any DNA added to it in the presence of all four types of

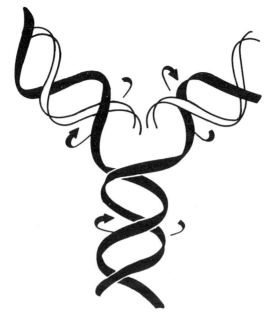

Fig. 10. The Y mechanism in the replication of DNA.

nucleoside 5′-triphosphates: deoxyadenosine, deoxythymidine, deoxycytidine, and deoxyguanosine triphosphates. The daughter chain grows by the stepwise interaction of deoxyribonucleoside 5′-triphosphate, with the 3′-hydroxyl group of the deoxyribose at the growing end of the daughter polynucleotide chain. Pyrophosphate is split off. The direction of synthesis is determined by the fact that each added nucleoside 5′-phosphate must bond to the 3′-hydroxyl of the preceding deoxyribose moiety. The base sequence, of course, will be complementary to the primer DNA. The DNA polymerase enzyme is very important to the specificity of the replication of the primer DNA. It must hold the backbone of the growing new chain against the backbone of the unwinding old chain in a position such that only the standard base pairs can form. The polymerase enzyme from *E. coli* has associated with it several nucleases that may play some role in the synthesis or replication of DNA.

STRUCTURE, FUNCTION, AND SYNTHESIS OF RNA

RNA is synthesized in a similar fashion to DNA, probably directly on the chromosomes and complementary in base sequence to DNA (Hurwitz and associates). The usual bases of RNA are adenine, guanine, uracil, and cytosine,

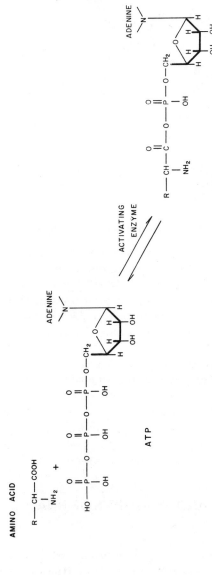

Fig. 11. Amino acid activation: formation of aminoacyl-AMP.

154

which form nucleosides with ribose. The nucleosides are linked with phosphoric acid as a $3'-5'$-phosphodiester, as is the case with DNA. The enzyme DNA-dependent RNA polymerase catalyzes the formation of RNA in the presence of DNA and all four ribonucleoside triphosphates. There are three classes of RNA's according to molecular weight: transfer RNA's found in the cell sap with a molecular weight range of 20,000 to 40,000; messenger RNA's with a molecular weight range of 200,000 or less, up to extremely large molecular weights; and ribosomal structural RNA's with a molecular weight of around 2,000,000.

The function of transfer RNA (tRNA) is to transfer the activated amino acids to the template (messenger) RNA on the ribosome. There are several different kinds of tRNA, at least one for each of the 20 different amino acids occurring naturally in protein. The amino acid is activated by a special activating enzyme, one for each amino acid called an aminoacyl synthetase. Energy is supplied by ATP. In the reaction shown in Figure 11, aminoacyl-AMP is formed and pyrophosphate is split off. The aminoacyl group of the aminoacyl-AMP is then transferred to the $2'$- or $3'$-hydroxyl of the terminal ribose of the tRNA to form aminoacyl-tRNA. AMP is split off (Fig. 12). This terminal ribose is part of the adenosine residue of the end group of transfer RNA. An ester apparently is formed between the aminoacyl group and the hydroxyl group of the ribose.

Messenger RNA (mRNA) carries the genetic information from the DNA of the gene to the site of protein synthesis, the ribosome. The rate of protein synthesis in a cell may be regulated by the rate of synthesis of mRNA, the amount of aminoacyl-tRNA for certain codons, protein factors involved in the binding of mRNA to the ribosome and in the attachment of aminoacyl-tRNA to

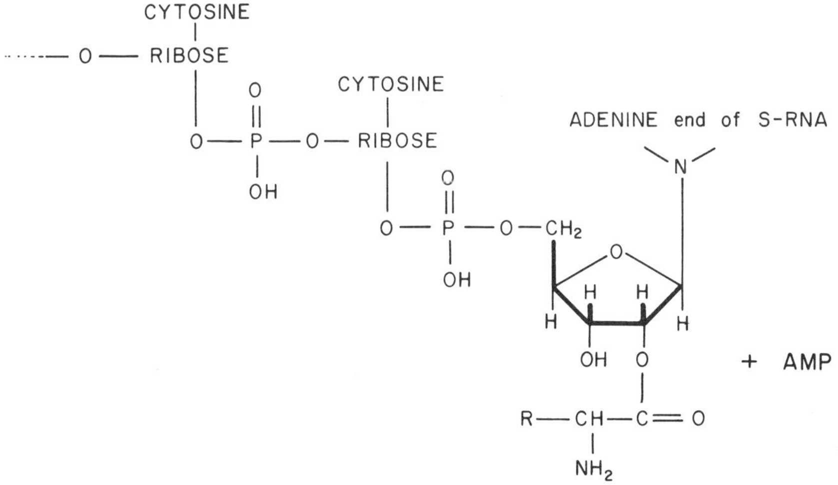

Fig. 12. Formation of aminoacyl-tRNA. The aminoacyl group from aminoacyl-AMP shown in Figure 11 has been transfered to the $2'$-hydroxyl of the terminal ribose of tRNA (sRNA).

the mRNA-ribosome, metabolic activity of the cell, availability of amino acids, or other processes. Some of the processes could be influenced by hormones. Messenger RNA turns over rapidly in bacterial cells but apparently is synthesized and degraded more slowly in mammalian cells. As mentioned previously, DNA-dependent RNA polymerase synthesizes mRNA against the base sequence of the template DNA. Thus, the base sequence of all the four ribonucleoside triphosphates previously mentioned is complementary in mRNA to that of the DNA. Many molecules of RNA may be synthesized against one molecule of DNA. In vivo it seems that only one strand of double-stranded DNA is copied, so that mRNA is single-stranded. Transcription of the DNA code to single-stranded mRNA may occur by means of a three-stranded DNA-RNA intermediate that does not involve unwinding of the DNA double helix. The RNA strand would dissociate readily after synthesis.

Ribosomal RNA and tRNA are apparently copied from parts of the DNA by RNA polymerase in similar fashion to the mRNA. The ribosomal structural RNA with the aid of protein factors bind the mRNA to form the translation template.

It is now possible to visualize a great deal about the structure of a gene. The nucleotide base sequence of an alanine transfer RNA isolated from yeast has been worked out by Holley and co-workers. Since the base sequence of one strand of the genetic DNA is complementary to the base sequence of the tRNA product, with some assumptions, the base sequence of DNA for the RNA isolated by Holley and associates can be deduced (Sonneborn). The nucleotide sequence of other tRNA's has been determined. For example, Dube and associates have worked out the complete sequence of N-formyl-methionyl-transfer RNA from *Escherichia coli*. This tRNA is part of the polypeptide initiation complex in bacteria.

PROTEIN BIOSYNTHESIS AND ENZYME ACTIVITY

The nucleotide base sequence of mRNA is a complementary polynucleotide of part of the base sequence of DNA. Thus, the complementary genetic code for the synthesis of a particular polypeptide or protein is carried by an mRNA attached to a ribosome. All ribosomes are made up of a larger (50S subunit) and smaller part (30S subunit) containing about equal parts of protein and structural RNA. The mRNA combines with the smaller parts of the ribosome. An initiating tRNA, such as formylmethionyl~$tRNA_F$ with the aid of protein-initiating factors, binds to this complex. The 50S ribosome subunit then binds. The ribosome is then activated for the synthesis of a particular protein depending on the code sequence of the bases of the mRNA attached as a template. A group of three adjacent nucleotide bases of the mRNA acts as a code for a single amino acid of the protein chain; the next three nucleotides act as a code for the next amino acid; and so on. Since there are four principal bases in nucleotides, 4^3, or 64, code words (codons) are possible for 20 naturally occurring amino acids. Thus, for several triplets, or codons, no amino acid corresponds, or several triplets must identify the same amino acid. The code of bases, or codon, for each amino acid has been ascertained. For example, Nirenberg and co-workers have shown that three uracils (UUU) in mRNA, complementary to three adenines (AAA) in chromosomal DNA, code for phenylalanine. Other base sequences for the 20 essential amino acids have been ascertained. The genetic code is given in Table 1.

Each amino acid is coded for by an mRNA triplet of nucleotides (codon) which has a specific sequence. AUG codes for methionine (Met), as shown, when it occurs in an internal position in a message. However, when it occurs in the 5′-terminal position of mRNA it specifies formyl methionine. Since the amino group is blocked with a formyl group, formyl methionine cannot form a peptide bond with the preceding amino acid. Thus, AUG functions as an initiation codon in the synthesis of polypeptides in bacteria.

The symbols N_1 (Amber), N_2 (Ochre), and N_3 represent three nonsense triplets, UAG, UAA, and UGA, which do not code for any amino acid. The

Table 1. THE GENETIC CODE

5′-Terminal Nucleotide	Middle Nucleotide				3′-Terminal Nucleotide
	U	C	A	G	
U	Phe	Ser	Tyr	Cys	U
	Phe	Ser	Tyr	Cys	C
	Leu	Ser	N2(Ochre)	N3	A
	Leu	Ser	N1(Amber)	Trp	G
C	Leu	Pro	His	Arg	U
	Leu	Pro	His	Arg	C
	Leu	Pro	Gln	Arg	A
	Leu	Pro	Gln	Arg	G
A	Ile	Thr	Asn	Ser	U
	Ile	Thr	Asn	Ser	C
	Ile	Thr	Lys	Arg	A
	Met	Thr	Lys	Arg	G
G	Val	Ala	Asp	Gly	U
	Val	Ala	Asp	Gly	C
	Val	Ala	Glu	Gly	A
	Val	Ala	Glu	Gly	G

nonsense triplets serve as terminator codons for growth of the polypeptide chain.

There are also different triplets coding for the same amino acid (degenerate codons). As many as six triplets can code for some amino acids, e.g., serine.

Much of the information on the regulation of the synthesis of DNA, RNA, and protein has been worked out with unicellular organisms. There is, however, good evidence that the code and the mechanism of protein synthesis are very similar in all organisms. Nevertheless, additional control mechanisms may have been added in multicellular organisms with the development of hormones that may regulate some component of mRNA synthesis, such as RNA polymerase, or a metabolic process essential to both replication of DNA and synthesis of mRNA.

The activated ribosome containing mRNA is ready to accept amino acids arranged in sequence according to the three-base codon sequence of mRNA, after formation of a chain initiation complex. In bacteria, a chain initiation complex, mRNA-ribosome-Fmet $\sim$ tRNA$_F$, begins the polypeptide sequence, in this case with formyl methionine (Fmet). Successive amino acids are brought to the ribosome by specific tRNA in the form of aminoacyl-tRNA, as described earlier. The aminoacyl-tRNA complexes become attached to the ribosomal particles in a sequence determined possibly by some complementary H-bonding relationship between the base code on the mRNA and the amino acid-specific molecule of tRNA. Since each tRNA molecule terminates in the same cytosine-cytosine-adenine trinucleotide sequence, specificity must reside in some other part of the tRNA. Each tRNA carries a code for recognizing the mRNA sequence for its amino acid. Since the base sequence of tRNA pairs to the base sequence of mRNA in a complementary fashion, the original base sequence of the DNA template of the gene is restored.

In translation of the genetic message from mRNA, the total length of the polypeptide synthesized is determined by the number of nucleotide triplets (codons) in the gene. AUG and probably GUG are initiating codons in bacteria, with the end of the message terminating by one of the nonsense codons, UAA (Ochre), UAG (Amber), and UGA (N_3). There are three processes involved: the formation of the chain initiation complex with mRNA, the incorporation of successive amino acids from incoming aminoacyl-tRNA with peptide bond formation and release of the tRNA, and finally chain termination with release of the polypeptide.

From studies of *Escherichia coli* systems it is apparent that formation of the chain initiation complex involves at least two separate steps: (1) binding of mRNA to the ribosome and (2) recognition of an AUG codon at the 5′ terminus of the mRNA by formyl methionyl$\sim$tRNA$_F$(Fmet$\sim$tRNA$_F$) with its attachment to form the complete initiation complex (mRNA-ribosome-Fmet$\sim$tRNA$_F$). There are also three protein factors (F_1, F_2, and F_3) isolated from *E. coli* ribosomes, involved in these steps. The binding of the mRNA to the ribosome requires F_3 and probably F_1. The attachment of Fmet~$tRNA_F$ to the ribosome-mRNA complex requires F_2. F_1 is also involved in the overall formation of the complete chain initiation complex. It is believed that all the proteins synthesized in bacteria are started with the same amino acid, formyl methionine. In mammalian cells and other multicellular cell systems, no doubt similar systems of chain initiation exist for amino acids other than formyl methionine.

Chain elongation can now proceed by successive incorporation of amino acids from aminoacyl tRNA according to the codon message of the mRNA. Studies with rat liver ribosomes have shown that guanosine triphosphate (GTP) and two protein factors obtained from the soluble fraction of liver homogenates are required. These protein factors have been called aminoacyl transferases I and II and probably represent different protein factors from those described for peptide chain initiation. The appropriate incoming aminoacyl-tRNA is bound to the next codon on mRNA according to its anticodon, and adjacent to the existing peptidyl-tRNA. Transferase I and GTP are involved in this binding to the ribosome. Synthesis of a new peptide bond occurs between the peptidyl-tRNA and the aminoacyl-tRNA, at the site occupied by the aminoacyl-tRNA. Synthesis of the peptide bond -C(=O)-NH- is carried out by ribosomes without transferase enzymes or GTP. The newly formed peptidyl-tRNA, now one amino acid longer, is transferred from the aminoacyl to the peptidyl site, under the influence of transferase II and GTP. This cycle repeats as the ribosome bound polypeptide chain is elongated one amino acid at a time.

Chain termination occurs when the codon sequence of nucleotides in mRNA ends in a nonsense triplet. As discovered in bacterial systems, UAA (Ochre), UAG (Amber), and UGA (N_3) do not code for any amino acids. Also required are two protein fractions called R1 and R2, which were isolated from the high-speed supernatant of homogenates of *E. coli*. The specificity of translation of the terminator codons is dependent on the R factors. R1 recognizes UAA and UAG; R2 recognizes UAA and UGA.

If the polypeptide is part of larger structural components of the cell, such as mitochondria or outer membranes, additional and unknown assembly mechanisms must occur. If the polypeptide chain (or chains) is an enzyme, either free in the cytoplasm or attached to a cell component, or as a structural and functional part of a cell component, then folding to some relatively stable structure undoubtedly occurs. There are several conformational changes in enzyme proteins that may influence function. Some may be random, but the changes are more likely to be induced by H-bonding groups, salt bonds, hydrophobic bonds, or by hormones, coenzymes, or substrates. The assembly of amino acids in a linear sequence constitutes the primary structure of the polypeptide. This linear sequence is formed by a bond between the amino group of one amino acid and the carboxyl group of another, called a peptide bond:

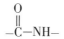

Genetic defects can occur in the primary structure, as, for example, in the hemoglobin of sickle-cell anemia. The chain, or a portion of the polypeptide chain, may coil helically around an axis to form an α helix. This coiling, held by H-bonding of the -C(=O)-NH-linkage of an amino acid residue to that of the third residue beyond, is called the secondary structure of the polypeptide. The distance between amino acid residues in an extended chain is about 3.5 angstroms, but is only 1.47 angstroms along the long axis of the α helix. Enzymes and biologically active polypeptides may have, in addition, a tertiary structure caused by folding of the polypeptide back upon itself; or two chains may be bonded by -S-S- linkages between cysteine residues, as with insulin. Certain enzymes and molecules, such as lactic and isocitric dehydrogenases and hemoglobin, may also form an aggregate of subunits or tertiary structures to produce a quatenary structure.

The tertiary structure of globular proteins, such as enzymes, may be largely determined by the sequence of certain amino acid residues in their polypeptide chains. A disulfide bridge between two cysteine residues, for example, is an important cross-linkage between two polypeptide chains or a folded chain that influences tertiary structure. Thus, a genetic aberration involving cysteine in the polypeptide chain could have important consequences in determining enzymatic function or activity. It is possible, however, in the case of certain rate-limiting enzymes of major metabolic pathways in mammalian cells, that the genetic code does not determine the final enzyme activity. Hormones may act as stimulators of the potential functional activity. For example, it has been suggested that ACTH might bind by H-bonding or electrostatic attraction of the free amino end of the polypeptide and the ε-amino groups of the lysine residues at positions 11, 15, 16, and 21 on the ACTH polypeptide to receptor groups on adrenal glucose-6-phosphate-dehydrogenase. This binding could cause a conformational change in the enzyme so that glucose-6-phosphate and nicotinamide adenine dinucleotide phosphate ($NADP^+$) are oriented for more efficient electron and H^+ transfer from substrate to the adenine nucleotide (McKerns, 1964). Other mechanisms of ACTH action are possible. Hydrogen bonding or electrostatic attraction of positively charged ACTH to negatively charged amino acids on the enzyme may increase the net positive charge around the substrate sites for both glucose-6-phosphate and $NADP^+$. Whatever the mechanism, ACTH causes a marked reduction of the apparent K_m for both substrates with a crystalline preparation of glucose-6-phosphate-dehydrogenase from the cow adrenal cortex (Criss and McKerns). The stimulation of this enzyme increases the activity of the pentose phosphate pathway and provides reducing equivalents as NADPH for steroid and fatty acid synthesis and provides phosphorylated ribose sugars for RNA and other nucleotide synthesis. This and other possible mechanisms of hormone actions are discussed in a separate chapter.

ABEL, P. Evidence for the universality of the genetic code. *Cold Spring Harbor Symp Quant Biol*, 29:185, 1964.

BISHOP, and SCHWEET, R. Synthesis of hemoglobin in a mixed cell-free system. *Biochim Biophys Acta*, 65:553, 1963.

CASKEY, C.T., BEAUDET, A., and NIRENBERG, M. RNA codons and protein synthesis. 15. Dissimilar responses of mammalian and bacterial transfer RNA fractions to messenger RNA codons. *J Molec Biol*, 37:99, 1968.

Cold Spring Harbor Symposia on Quantitative Biology. Long Island, New York, Cold Spring Harbor Laboratory of Quantitative Biology, 1968, Vol 31.

CRICK, F.H.C. The biochemistry of genetics. Plenary Sessions, *Sixth Internat Congr Biochem*, 33:109, 1964.

—— and WATSON, J.D.H. Molecular structure of nucleic acids. *Nature (London)*, 171:737, 1953.

CRISS, W.E. and McKERNS, K.W. Activation of cow adrenal glucose-6-phosphate dehydrogenase by adrenocorticotropin. *Biochemistry*, 7:2364, 1968.

DUBE, S.K., MARCKER, K.A., CLARK, B.F.C., and CORY, S. Nucleotide sequence of N-formyl-methionyl-transfer RNA. *Nature (London)*, 218:232, 1968.

FESSENDEN, J.M., and MOLDAVE, K. Studies on aminoacyl transfer from soluble ribonucleic acid to ribosomes. *J Biol Chem*, 238:1479, 1963.

FRANKLIN, R.E., and GOSLING, R.G. Molecular configuration in sodium thymonucleate. *Nature (London)*, 171:740, 1953.

GAREN, A. Sense and nonsense in the genetic code. *Science*, 160:149, 1968.

GOODMAN, H.M., and RICH, A. Formation of a DNA-soluble RNA hybrid and its relation to the origin, evolution, and degeneracy of soluble RNA. *Proc Nat Acad Sci USA*, 48:2101, 1962.

HECHT, L.I., STEPHENSION, M.L., and ZAMECNIK, P.C. Binding of amino acids to the end group of a soluble ribonucleic acid. *Proc Nat Acad Sci USA*, 45:505, 1959.

HOLLEY, R.W., APGAR, J., EVERETT, G.A., MADISON, J.T., MARQUISEE, M., MERRILL, S.H., PENSWICK, J.R., and ZAMIR, A. Structure of a ribonucleic acid. *Science*, 147:1462, 1965.

HURWITZ, J., FURTH, J.J., ANDERS, M., ORTIZ, P.J., and AUGUST, J.T. The enzymatic incorporation of ribonucleotides into RNA and the role of DNA. *Cold Spring Harbor Symp Quant Biol*, 26:91, 1961.

IBUKI, F., and MOLDAVE, K. Evidence for the enzymatic binding of aminoacyl transfer ribonucleic acid to rat liver ribosomes. *J Biol Chem*, 243:791, 1968.

IWASAKI, K., SABOL, S., WAHBA, A.J., and OCHOA, S. Translation of the genetic message. VII. Role of initiation factors in formation of the chain initiation complex with *Escherichia coli* ribosomes. *Arch Biochem*, 125:542, 1968.

JACOB, F., and MONOD, J. Genetic regulatory mechanisms in the synthesis of proteins. *J Molec Biol*, 3:318, 1961.

KORNBERG, A. Enzymatic synthesis of DNA. *Ciba Lectures Microbiol Biochem.* New York, John Wiley & Sons, Inc., 1962, Vol. 5, p. 1.

LODISH, H.F. Bacteriophage f2 RNA: Control of translation and gene order. *Nature (London)*, 220:345, 1968.

MARKER, K., and SANGER, F. N-formyl-methionyl-S-RNA. *J Molec Biol.* 8:835, 1964.

McKERNS, K.W. Genetic, biochemical and hormonal mechanisms in the regulation of uterine metabolism. *In* Wynn, R.M., ed. *Cellular Biology of the Uterus.* New York, Appleton-Century-Crofts, 1967, Chap. 5.

—— Mechanism of action of adrenocorticotropic hormone through activation of glucose-6-phosphate dehydrogenase. *Biochim Biophys Acta,* 90:357, 1964.

MONOD, J., CHANGEUX, J.-P., and JACOB, F. Allosteric proteins and cellular control systems. *J Molec Biol,* 6:306, 1963.

NIRENBERG, M.W., LEDER, P., BERNFIELD, M., BRIMACOMBE, R., TRUPIN, J., ROTTMAN, F., and O'NEAL, C. RNA code words and protein synthesis. VII. On the general nature of the RNA code. *Proc Nat Acad Sci USA,* 53:1161, 1965.

—— and MATTHAEI, J.H. Comparison of ribosomal and soluble *E. coli* systems incorporating amino acids into protein. *Fifth Internat Congr Biochem (Moscow),* 1961, p. 102.

SCOLNICK, E., TOMPKINS, R., CASKEY, T., and NIRENBERG, M. Release factors differing in specificity for terminator codons. *Proc Nat Acad Sci USA,* 61:768, 1968.

SKOGERSON, L., and MOLDAVE, K. Evidence for the role of aminoacyltransferase II in peptidyl transfer ribonucleic acid translocation. *J Biol Chem,* 243:5361, 1968.

SONNEBORN, T.M. Nucleotide sequence of a gene: First complete specification. *Science,* 148:1410, 1965.

SPIEGELMAN, S., and HAYASHI, M. The present status of the transfer of genetic information and its control. *Cold Spring Harbor Symp Quant Biol,* 28:161, 1963.

STENT, G.S. Replication of DNA. *In Molecular Biology of Bacterial Viruses.* San Francisco, W.H. Freeman & Co, Publishers, 1963.

STEWART, C.D., ANAND, S.R., and BESSMAN, M.J. Studies on the synthesis of deoxyribonucleic acid. II. Studies with biologically active templates and the stimulation of synthesis by oligonucleotides. *J Biol Chem,* 243:5319, 1968.

WATSON, J.D.H., and CRICK, F.H.C. Genetical implications of the structure of deoxyribonucleic acid. *Nature (London),* 171:964, 1953.

WEISS, S.B., and NAKAMATO, T. On the participation of DNA in RNA biosynthesis. *Proc Nat Acad Sci USA,* 47:694, 1961.

WILKINS, M.F.H., and RANDLE, J.T. Crystallinity in sperm heads: Molecular structure of nucleoprotein in vivo. *Biochim Biophys Acta,* 10:192, 1953.

WOESE, C.R. *The Genetic Code.* New York, Harper & Row, 1967.

11

Principles of the Mechanism of Hormone Action

Some current concepts of hormone action will be discussed in a general fashion in this chapter for the purpose of identifying some basic questions involved in the role of hormones as regulators of cellular function. There are several possible ways in which hormones could modify the activity and stimulate the growth of cells of their target tissues. Many of the recent studies on the mechanisms of hormone action have been directed toward the concept that hormones affect gene action on the transcription level (DNA-directed RNA synthesis). Some investigators have also suggested that hormones regulate at the translational level, and affect the rate of protein synthesis from mRNA.

Jacob and Monod demonstrated in bacterial systems that substrates were able to induce the synthesis of specific enzymes concerned with their metabolism. They suggested that the amino acid sequence of protein enzymes is controlled by structural genes through the synthesis of mRNA. The rate of synthesis of mRNA, in turn, is said to be controlled by so-called operator genes. In this system, the activity of the genes may be regulated by repressor substrates which block gene action. Jacob and Monod presented evidence that these repressors are inactivated by certain metabolites which then act as inducers of enzyme synthesis. Since substrate inducers in single-cell organisms were presumably around long before hormones, it seemed only natural to consider that in more specialized organisms hormones might act either to increase the level of the substrate inducer, or by some mechanism directly affect an aspect of transcription or translation.

Thus, the control function of many hormones, especially steroid hormones, has been related to the concept that the hormone directly or indirectly modifies the genome template to increase the synthesis of some or all of the messenger RNA. That is to say, the hormones could increase the capacity of the chromatin to act as a template for DNA-dependent RNA polymerase. This effect presumably precedes the increase in the rate of formation of ribosomal precursor particles and the general increase in nuclear and cytoplasmic synthesis of protein.

Jensen has shown that after the administration of various radioactive steroids to animals, the radioactive steroid is rapidly picked up by what one would expect to be the target tissue for the hormone. For example, the administration of H^3-estradiol to the immature rat leads to a rapid uptake and retention of the hormone by the uterus, vagina, and anterior pituitary. In the case of the uterus, most of the radioactive estradiol was found to locate in the nucleus, and nuclear RNA synthesis is stimulated as one of the earliest effects of the administration of the hormone. The analysis of chromatin extracted from the nucleus shows that this consists of DNA, acidic proteins, and basic proteins of high molecular weight, such as histones. Histones are rich in the basic amino acids, arginine and lysine. The histones have been suspected to be gene regulators by combining with DNA through ionic linkages between anionic phosphate groups of DNA and cationic groups of the basic amino acids.

Recent experiments have demonstrated that at least part of the protein material of the chromatin is a receptor for estradiol and binds it with a high affinity and specificity. A working hypothesis has suggested that either the combination of estradiol with an acidic nuclear protein combines with the histones, or else the protein-estradiol complex has some stimulatory effect on DNA-dependent RNA synthesis. This same mechanism of action has been suggested to account for the regulation of the growth of the prostate by androgens; the regulation of the synthesis of a protein concerned in stimulating what might be an energy-dependent transport of sodium out of the epithelial cell of the frog bladder by aldosterone; the effect of glucocorticoids in inducing enzyme synthesis in the liver; the effect of the insect hormone ecdysone in regulating the transition of insect larvae to pupae; and the action of many other hormones.

From necessity, most of the theories as to the complete mechanism of hormone action are deductive. That is to say, even if nuclear RNA synthesis is activated very early after the administration of estrogen, the exact mechanism of this effect has not been proven. Implicit in many of the ideas of hormone action is the concept that genes are blocked or repressed and control of transcription is achieved by specific inducers which de-repress. This is by no means proven, nor is it clear what these possible repressors might be.

Other fundamental concepts concerning cell regulation are not understood. For example, after the fertilization of the mammalian ovum, its implantation, and during the growth of the fetus, there is the problem of how tissue differentiation is achieved. Do all cells, for example, in a multicellular organism contain the same sequences of nucleotide triplets in DNA with specificity achieved by permanent blocking of part of the genome; or as cells differentiate during fetal growth, do regulators allow only certain sequences of nucleotide triplets in DNA to be replicated? In other words, does a specialized cell contain only the nucleotide sequences in DNA that are ultimately expressed as proteins unique to its cellular function? Even if a differentiated cell does contain only genes relative to its specific function, are these genes only capable of directing the synthesis of RNA when they are de-repressed by substrates, hormones, or other regulators?

It is also possible that DNA can direct the synthesis of RNA relative to metabolic activity and to the availability of adequate purine and pyrimidine triphosphates. This control could be in terms of regulating the metabolic activity of the cell by the provisions of compounds such as 5-phosphoribosyl pyrophosphate, which a hormone could conceivably control by regulating metabolic pathways such as the pentose phosphate pathway. Another possibility would be that increased substrates derived from hormonal stimulation could act as inducers of RNA synthesis.

Future research no doubt will determine whether the genetic material of all cells in the organism, at least within one species, contains the same sequence of nucleotide triphosphates in the nucleus. If this were the case, then it would be necessary to determine as well how unique specificity was achieved for specialized cells. This could be accomplished by controlling the start of the read-off for synthesis of a particular mRNA and terminating the sequence by various initiators and terminators. In such a case one would have to postulate that transcription of DNA could start at a specific nucleotide triplet in the DNA nucleotide sequence under the control of an initiator, with the end of read-off controlled by a specific terminator. As yet no such regulatory factors for transcription of DNA have been discovered. However, initiating factors have been described for translation of mRNA in ribosomes from *Escherichia coli.* It is conceivable that hormones may have some effect in regulating the synthesis of specific protein factors involved in the initiation of polypeptide synthesis. This is unproven. It is popular to suppose that transcription of certain nucleotide sequences in DNA is blocked by repressors such as histones, and substrates or hormones unmask the DNA in some fashion. This implies, for any one cell, thousands of nucleotide sequences, each sequence utilized for transcription of only one unique mRNA, used in turn, for translation of one polypeptide chain. This would also apply to the synthesis of ribosomal RNA synthesized from DNA in the nucleolus and to the synthesis of various tRNA's. Some economy could be realized by assembly of various groupings of polypeptide chains into specialized structural or enzyme proteins. There would seem to be adequate nucleotides in the DNA of vertebrates to have unique sequences for these purposes. In addition, there may be many copies of these sequences incorporated into the genome.

The experiments of Gurdon and Ulinger are interesting and relevant to some of these possibilities. These workers removed nuclei from the interstitial epithelial cells of the gut of *Xenopus laevis* tadpoles and transplanted them into unfertilized eggs of frogs that were enucleated by ultraviolet irradiation. Many of the nuclear-transplanted embryos reached advanced development stages, some to adult frogs. The implication from these experiments is that even specialized cells contain in their nucleus the complete genetic information for any cell function. Specialized function would then have to be the suppression of irrelevant genetic information. In addition, transcription or translation relative to the specialized function of the cell would have to be further modulated by hormones and other inducers.

In regard to the mechanism of action of trophic hormones, it has been postulated that thyroid-stimulating hormone, luteinizing hormones, adrenocorticotropic hormone, and others stimulate a specific adenyl cyclase in their target tissue, leading to an increase in $3',5'$-AMP. This latter compound is suggested as a mediator of the hormone action. In addition to whatever effect $3',5'$-AMP has in converting phosphorylase b to the active enzyme (see Figure 2, Chapter 3) it has also been implicated as an inducer of DNA-directed RNA synthesis. Thus, for the trophic hormones, mechanisms have been evoked similar to those described for steroid hormones, except that $3',5'$-AMP is proposed to act as a second messenger for gene activation. Again, if true, the exact mechanism is unknown.

An alternate suggestion to the idea of gene activation by de-repression is that trophic hormones stimulate an increased rate of reduction of $NADP^+$ and an increased rate of metabolism of glucose-6-phosphate by the pentose phosphate cycle (see Figure 9, Chapter 2). This could be accomplished through unique species of glucose-6-phosphate dehydrogenase having receptor groups for their activating hormones. These receptor groups are different from the substrate binding groups. For example, glucose-6-phosphate dehydrogenase purified from the adrenal cortex has been shown to have complementary H-bonding groups or negatively charged amino groups that electrostatically attract the free amino end and the ϵ-amino groups of the lysine residues at positions 11, 15, 16, and 21 on the ACTH polypeptide. ACTH reduces the apparent K_m for $NADP^+$ and glucose-6-phosphate, either by inducing a conformational change in the enzyme that makes the active center more accessible, or by increasing the net positive charge around the substrate sites on the enzyme.

Unless stimulated, glucose-6-phosphate dehydrogenase, and consequently the pentose phosphate pathway, may have little activity at the cellular levels of glucose-6-phosphate and NADP$^+$. An assessment of the activity of the pathway in the tissues relative to the amount of glucose-6-phosphate metabolized by glycolysis may have little validity, unless the marked change induced by hormones is considered. Increasing levels of glucose-6-phosphate and NADP$^+$ increase the rate of reduction of NADP$^+$ by purified glucose-6-phosphate dehydrogenase in vitro. The addition of one mole of ACTH to one mole of enzyme further increases these rates until maximum velocity is achieved. Similarly, the addition of glucose-6-phosphate and NADP$^+$ to homogenates of whole adrenal tissue stimulates steroidogenesis. When ACTH is added, the reactions are stimulated further. This effect has been interpreted by some as evidence that trophic hormones and NADPH affect steroidogenesis by different mechanisms. Actually, from studies on crystalline glucose-6-phosphate dehydrogenase, it is apparent that the extra increase in rate is due to changes in substrate-binding affinities in the enzymes, induced by ACTH. In addition to increasing the supply of reducing equivalents, ACTH could provide ribose sugars for synthesis of nucleotides required in the synthesis of RNA and DNA.

As shown in Figure 6, Chapter 10, orotate and 5-phospho-D-ribosyl pyrophosphate (5-PRPP) form orotidine-5'-phosphate under the direction of the enzyme orotidine-5'-phosphate pyrophosphorylase. Orotidine-5'-phosphate can be converted to the parent pyrimidine compound, uridine-5'-phosphate. The rate-limiting reaction to the formation of pyrimidines and possibly to purine triphosphates may be the availability of 5-PRPP derived during the metabolism of glucose-6-phosphate by the pentose phosphate pathway, as shown in Figure 9, Chapter 2. It has been demonstrated that ACTH, by stimulating glucose-6-phosphate dehydrogenase and thus the pentose phosphate pathway, increases the rate of formation of 5-PRPP from glucose-6-phosphate in high-speed supernatant fractions prepared from adrenal cortex. In the presence of added orotate, the rate of formation of uridine-5'-phosphate was increased. These effects of the hormone occur, therefore, in the absence of any nuclear DNA or ribosomal RNA.

Luteinizing hormone and human chorionic gonadotrophin were also found to stimulate the rate of reduction of NADP$^+$ by ovarian glucose-6-phosphate dehydrogenase and to increase the synthesis of uridine-5'-phosphate in a similar system of high-speed supernatant fractions prepared from rat ovaries. The rats were pretreated with pregnant mare serum gonadotropin. These experiments suggest that both the immediate synthetic function of certain endocrine tissues, as well as the rate of synthesis of RNA and eventually cell replication, could be controlled by trophic hormones at the level of glucose-6-phosphate dehydrogenase. (McKerns 1968, 1969; Criss and McKerns).

Other theories in regard to ACTH action suggest that the conversion of cholesterol to 5-pregnenolone by mitochondrial enzymes is directly stimulated. This could occur either by activation of 20α-hydroxylase, an increase in synthesis of a rate-limiting enzyme by increased translation from an mRNA, or by other mechanisms. Even if hormones are able to stimulate the activity of certain enzymes that are rate-limiting to function, there may be other regulators of transcription and translation independent of hormone control. With many tissues, however, it is apparent that hormone regulation is essential to cell function and replication.

Various classes of hormones, of course, may regulate cell function by different mechanisms. Certain hormones, such as insulin, may increase permeability of cell membranes to substrates. Furthermore, the same hormone may have different effects in different tissues. Estradiol stimulates growth of the endometrium of the uterus, but may inhibit the synthesis of follicle-stimulating hormone in the anterior pituitary. Various other steroids have been shown to be inhibitors of enzyme reactions in various tissues. For example, estrogens, androgens, pregnenolone, progesterone, and thyronine compounds are competitive inhibitors of $NADP^+$ binding to glucose-6-phosphate dehydrogenase. Some of these steroids could conceivably be regulators of cell function in certain tissues, for example, the adrenal cortex. Glucocorticoids are also antianabolic, in that they inhibit protein synthesis in certain tissues.

In addition to the effect that hormones have in regulating the function of existing cells, they also stimulate growth of certain of their target tissues. Among other things, cell replication involves duplication of the genetic material. Mechanisms of intracellular initiation and synthesis of DNA are little understood. Certainly the role of hormones at the molecular level in DNA replication is obscure because of this. Proteins from the nucleus may relax or uncover double stranded DNA to provide a small region, of single stranded DNA. This region could be available for base pairing with small oligonucleotide initiators. With DNA polymerase and nucleotide substrates, DNA synthesis could proceed from the $3'$-hydroxy group of the oligonucleotide. As the DNA uncoils, unidirectional synthesis of both daughter strands of DNA could proceed to the end of the template or until another bound polynucleotide is encountered. These concepts have been discussed by Steuart et al.

Tremendous progress has been made in molecular biology in the discovery of the chemical basis of heredity, in the structure of the gene, and in the operation of the genetic code. Obviously these achievements have made more urgent the need for further research leading toward full understanding of the mechanisms that control cell function and replication. Some of the experimental approaches to these problems have been described briefly in preceding chapters, and the general problems and the general direction of research have been alluded to.

BRANSOME, E.D., and CADWGAN, C.E. Cytoplasmic RNA synthesis in adrenal: rapid, selective stimulation by adrenocorticotropic hormone (ACTH). *Life Sci*, 7:1009, 1968.

BRITTEN, R.J., and KOHNE, D.E. Repeated sequences in DNA. *Science*, 161:529, 1968.

CRISS, W.E. and McKERNS, K.W. Activation of cow adrenal glucose-6-phosphate dehydrogenase by adrenocorticotropin. *Biochemistry*, 7:2364, 1968.

DAVIS, W.W., and GARREN, L.D. On the mechanism of action of adrenocorticotropic hormone. *J Biol Chem*, 243:5153, 1968.

DeLANGE, R.J., FAMBROUGH, D.M., SMITH, E.L., and BONNER, J. Calf and pea histone IV: II. The complete amino acid sequence of calf thymus histone IV; presence of ϵ-N-acetyllsine. *J Biol Chem*, 244:319, 1969.

GURDON, J.B., and UHLINGER, V. "Fertile" intestinal nuclei. *Nature (London)*, 210:1240, 1966.

HAMILTON, T.H. Control by estrogen of genetic transcription and translation. *Science*, 161:649, 1968.

IWASAKI, K., SABOL, S., WAHBA, A.J., and OCHOA, S. Translation of the genetic message. VII. Role of initiation factors in formation of the chain initiation complex with *Echerichia coli* ribosomes. *Arch Biochem*, 125:542, 1968.

JACOB, F., and MONOD, J. Genetic regulatory mechanisms in the synthesis of proteins. *J Molec Biol*, 3:318, 1961.

JENSEN, E.V. Metabolic fate of sex hormones in target tissues with regard to tissue specificity. *Proceedings of the Second International Congress of Endocrinology*. Amsterdam, Excerpta Medica Foundation, Ser. No. 83, 1964, pp. 420-433.

——Estrogen binding substances of target tissues. *Proceedings of the Third International Congress of Endocrinology*, Mexico City. Amsterdam, Excerpta Medica Foundation, 1968.

KARLSON, P., and SEKERIS, C.E. Biochemical mechanisms of hormone action. *Acta Endocr. (Kobenhavn)*, 53:505, 1966.

KING, R.J., and GORDON, J. The association of $[6,7\text{-}^3\text{H}]$ oestradiol with a nuclear protein. *J. Endocr*, 39:533, 1967.

LANGAN, T.A. Histone phosphorylation: stimulation by adenosine $3',5'$-monophosphate. *Science*, 162:579, 1968.

LIAO, S., and LIN, A.H. Prostatic nuclear chromatin: an effect of testosterone on the synthesis of ribonucleic acid rich in cytidylyl $(3',5')$ guanosine. *Proc Nat Acad Sci USA*, 57:379, 1967.

MARUSHIGE, K., BRUTLAG, D., and BONNER, J. Properties of chromosomal nonhistone protein of rat liver. *Biochemistry*, 7:3149, 1968.

McKERNS, K.W. The regulation of adrenal function by estrogens and other hormones. *Biochim Biophys Acta*, 71:710, 1963.

—— Genetic, biochemical, and hormonal mechanisms in the regulation of uterine metabolism. *In* Wynn, R.M., ed. *Cellular Biology of the Uterus*. New York, Appleton-Century-Crofts, 1967, Chap. 5.

—— ,ed. *Functions of the Adrenal Cortex*. New York, Appleton-Century-Crofts, 1968.

—— Mechanisms of ACTH regulation of the adrenal cortex. *In* McKerns, K.W., ed. *Functions of the Adrenal Cortex*. New York, Appleton-Century-Crofts, 1968, Vol. 1, Chap. 12.

—— , ed. *The Gonads*. New York, Appleton-Century-Crofts, 1969.

——Studies on the regulation of ovarian function by gonadotrophins. *In*

McKerns, K.W., ed. *The Gonads.* Part 1: Functions of the Ovaries. New York, Appleton-Century-Crofts, 1969, Chap. 6.

MONOD, J., CHANGEUX, J.P., and JACOB, F. Allosteric proteins and cellular control systems. *J Molec Biol,* 6:306, 1963.

NICOLETTE, J.A., LEMAHIEU, M.A., and MUELLER, G.C. A role of estrogens in the regulation of RNA polymerase in surviving rat uteri. *Biochim Biophys Acta,* 166:403, 1968.

O'MALLEY, B.W., ARONOW, A., PEACOCK, A.C., and DINGMAN, C.W. Estrogen-dependent increase in transfer RNA during differentiation of the chick oviduct. *Science,* 162:567, 1968.

PUCA, G.A., and BRESCIANI, F. Receptor molecule for oestrogens from rat uterus. *Nature (London),* 218:967, 1968.

ROBISON, G.A., BUTCHER, R.W., and SUTHERLAND, E.W. Cyclic AMP. *Ann. Rev. Biochem,* 37:149, 1968.

SEGAL, S.J., and SCHER, W. Estrogens, nucleic acids, and protein synthesis in uterine metabolism. *In* Wynn, R.M., ed. *Cellular Biology of the Uterus.* New York, Appleton-Century-Crofts, 1967, Chap. 6.

STEUART, C.D., ANAND, S.R., and BESSMAN, M.J. Studies on the synthesis of deoxyribonucleic acid. II. Studies with biologically active templates and the stimulation of synthesis of oligonucleotides. *J Biol Chem,* 243:5319, 1968.

TAUNTON, O.D., ROTH, J., and PASTAN, I. Studies on the adrenocorticotropic hormone-activated adenyl cyclase of a functional adrenal tumor. *J Biol Chem,* 244:247, 1969.

TOMPKINS, G. Hormones and genes: Transcriptional effect. *Proceedings of the Third International Congress of Endocrinology,* Mexico City. Amsterdam, Excerpta Medica Foundation, 1968.

TRACHEWSKY, D., and SEGAL, S.J. Differential synthesis of ribonucleic acid in uterine nuclei: Evidence for selective gene transcription induced by estrogens. *European J Biochem,* 4:279, 1968.

VOGEL, H.J., and VOGEL, R.H. Regulation of protein synthesis. *Ann Rev Biochem,* 36:519, 1967.

WYATT, G.R., and TATA, J.R. The hybridization capacity of ribonucleic acid produced during hormone action. *Biochem J,* 109:253, 1968.

INDEX

DNA
  genetic material, 145
  helix, 149
  as polynucleotide molecule, 149-151
  replication, 151-153
  transcription, effect of repressors, 165
DNA-dependent RNA polymerase, 152, 156
Double helix, DNA, 151-153

Electron flow
  in mitochondria and microsomes, 26-29
  from NADPH, 27
Electron-transport chain, steroid hydroxylation, 27
Energy-dependent transhydrogenase, steroid hydroxylation, 27
Energy metabolism, in adrenal cortex, 17
Enolase, 46
Epinephrine, phosphorylase a effect, 33
Estradiol, metabolic products, 100
Estrane, parent compound, 5
Estrogen
  biosynthesis, from androgens, 17
  effect on fatty acid synthesis, 138
  urinary excretion, 99-100
Extramitochondrial reducing equivalents, in steroid hydroxylations, 27-28

FAD reduction, in fatty acid oxidation, 124
Fascicular zone, steroid synthesis in, 11
Fatty acid
  biosynthetic systems, 110
  catabolism, 121
  cytoplasmic biosynthesis, palmitic acid, 111-113
  desaturation, 120-121
  metabolism
    control, 133
    ratio oxidized: reduced coenzymes, 135
  mitochondrial synthesis, 119-120
  oxidation
    effect on pyruvate metabolism, 48
    in energy production, 139
  β-oxidation reactions, 123
  saturated, unsaturated, 108

Fatty acid (cont.)
  synthesis
    influence of diet, 134
    pentose cycle dehydrogenases, 116
    role of carnitine, 136
    sources of carbon, 111
    sources of reductive hydrogen, 116
    unsaturated, 120
  synthetases, 118
Fatty acyl-CoA, dehydrogenases in liver mitochondria, 123
Fetal-placental steroid relationships, 88-91
Fructoaldolase, 46
Fructose-1,6-diphosphatase, 47

Gene
  action, hormone effect on, 163
  function, summary, 146
  as mRNA template, 145
Genetic code, 156-158
Genetic expression, hormone modification, 145
Genome template, hormone effect on, 163-164
Glomerular zone, steroid synthesis in, 13-15
Glucagon, phophorylase a effect, 33
Glucocorticoid
  action on lymphocytes, 54
  effect in gluconeogenesis, 32
Glucocorticoids and immune response, 51-55
Gluconeogenesis, 33
  pathways of substrate metabolism, 49-51
  pyruvate to glucose, 37
  regulation of, 36-37
  unidirectional enzymes in, 43-48
Gluconeogenesis and glycolysis in liver, summary of, 50-51
Gluconeogenic enzymes, 43
Glucose homeostasis, 36-37
Glucose metabolism, in adrenal cortex, 20
Glucose-6-phosphatase, 47
Glucose-6-phosphate metabolism
  in endocrine tissues, 20
  by pentose phosphate pathway, 22
Glutamate-oxalacetate transaminase, 39
D-Glyceraldehyde-3-phosphate dehydrogenase, 46
Glutamate-pyruvate transamination, 39